Dedicated to the Scribbling Women of CBHP

A Healing Journey

A Healing Journey

WRITING TOGETHER
THROUGH BREAST CANCER

Sharon Bray, Ed.D.

AMHERST WRITERS & ARTISTS PRESS

2004

Copyright © 2004 by Sharon Bray

FIRST EDITION

Published by
Amherst Writers & Artists Press
Box 1076
Amherst, MA 01004

ISBN 0-941895-29-7

Designed by Barbara Werden
Set in Bembo with Amethyst display

06 07 / 4 3 2

CONTENTS

Preface   ix

Acknowledgments   xiii

Introduction: The Call to Writing   1

1   Creating A Healing Environment   6

2   When Writing Is Healing: What the Research Tells Us   18

3   From Campfires to Writing Groups: The Healing Power of Story   30

4   Opening Up: The First Experience in an Amherst Writers & Artists Workshop   39

5   A Personal Journey of Writing and Healing   46

6   From Pilot to Program   54

7   Writing Together: The Scribbling Women of CBHP   68

8   When One Loss Begets the Memory of Another   80

9   Writing as Sanctuary   88

10   The Valley of the Shadow of Death   107

11   On Being a Writing Group Leader   124

Epilogue   135

Appendix: Selected Writing Exercises   137

References and Resources   143

PREFACE

I am grateful to have been asked to write the preface to this book. Before I read it, perhaps because I know Sharon Bray personally and know the artistic discipline she embraces as writer and leader of writing workshops, I expected it to be moving. Because I am aware of her study of psychology, healing, and various approaches to writing and spirituality, I expected the work to be wisely connected to contemporary writers and healers whose work most informs her own. It is all of that. What I did not foresee was that the voices of women in these pages would enable me to look directly at my own cancer experience and deepen my own healing journey.

A Healing Journey: Writing Together through Breast Cancer is a book by, about, and for women who live with breast cancer, and for those who care about them. It is also for professionals in the healing arts who increasingly are looking to writing as a healing methodology. And it is for writers, teachers of writing, and workshop leaders who want to know how effectively to use writing as a healing practice with persons experiencing life-threatening illnesses.

Bray has brought together in her own life and in her healing practice the primary disciplines of the Amherst Writers & Artists (AWA) writing workshop method, and the research of medical pioneers Dr. James W. Pennebaker, Dr. David Spiegel, and others. The AWA method gives her a structured and disciplined approach to keep a writing group functioning as a supportive community. Pennebaker's and Spiegel's research underlie and confirm her conviction that writing together without judgment, and sharing that writing with others who receive it with acceptance and affirmation, actually does bring about healing in the human body. From them, too, she is strengthened in her understanding of the importance of story. She says:

> Translating our distress into story allows us the perspective to forget or move beyond it. Writing our stories certainly gives us a chance to live life twice, but more importantly, it gives us an opportunity to make sense out of our lives, understand how we have changed, or what we have learned from major life events. Healing is also learning, and the retrospective look that allows us to find the meaning in our life's experiences is key to reaping healing benefits from writing.

Bray gives us in these pages very human stories of life and death. On one level, this book is her own story—how one woman responded to her own breast cancer by study and experimentation until she created a healing methodology for other women with cancer diagnoses. It is also a practical guide to writing workshops for persons with life-threatening illness, including practices that keep groups supportive, medical theory, the boundary between writing groups and group therapy, and sample writing exercises.

I especially appreciate Bray's clear distinction between writing-workshop-as-healing-environment and group therapy. To me, this is one of the most important contributions of this book to the growing understanding of the potential for healing through writing together in supportive environments. Amherst Writers & Artists has insisted throughout its history that writing is both an art form and a healing practice. Using it as a healing force for both personal and societal ills does not compromise its integrity as an art form. Put more directly, writing can escape the ivory halls and the dusty canon. It can ride city buses as it has done since a brilliant dancer, Frances Balter, first put "Poetry on the Buses" in Philadelphia. Not only can genius in writing *ride,* however. It can be born in housing projects and walk the streets of ghettos; it can come into being in men's prisons and in elementary schools. As Sharon Bray absolutely demonstrates here, it can be created between women who journey with cancer. Writing can do those things and not be compromised as art. Art belongs to the human spirit, and genius erupts wherever the human spirit reaches out to exult, to rage, or to tell the story of the healed or healing heart.

Within Bray's central narrative, as often happens in good writing, she gives us many stories, in her own words and in the words of women who wrote with her. Her own cancer story caused me to examine my reaction to a cancer diagnosis. She describes her visit to the doctor, how she cheerily receives and responds to the news he gives her, and only the next day is suddenly stunned:

> "John," I called to my husband. "He said carcinoma, didn't he?"
> My husband nodded.
> "That's cancer," I exclaimed, my eyes wide with fear and sudden understanding.
> John nodded again, "Yes, that's cancer."

Bray does not spare her reader the complexity of either the personal or the communal experience of writing together through cancer. For example, a poem written in workshop invites us to feel "the vulnerability and complex emotions of a woman [Karen Jandorf] who lost both breasts to cancer":

> If you touch my chest, you will feel my heart in your hand.
> It is that close to the surface.
> All its protective covering has been taken away.

As we are given access to the intimate life stories of women who experience breast cancer, our understanding of the need for supportive writing community becomes clear. In response to that need, this book is good news. In these pages, medical science and the art of writing embrace one another, and what is born is beautiful. Often the greatest genius simply reveals a truth that we already know in our hearts. Here, in the words of women struggling with cancer, is this truth: when we open our life stories to one another truly and deeply, and those stories are received with loving acceptance, healing happens.

PAT SCHNEIDER

ACKNOWLEDGMENTS

The beginnings of this book are inextricably bound up in a group of women who, as they discovered their voices and courage in the midst of cancer, became "The Scribbling Women of CBHP." Many of their stories, poems, and prose pieces appear in this book. Some have won the battle with this dreadful disease and moved on; others still write with me at the Community Breast Health Project; others have suffered recurrences and left us a legacy of story as testimony to their lives. The many women who have been part of the Scribbling Women of CBHP will always be in my memory, but a particular thank you goes to a small group of women who were so instrumental in helping me think about this book, and whose work appears within its pages: Jean Allington, Judy Finney, Irena Olender, Sheree Kirby, Carolyn Schuk, Candice Michel, Karen Jandorf, Karen Usatine, Clarissa Magno Cua, Ceci Martinez, Margaret Prien, Marcia Davis-Cannon, Neli Stascausky, Bernadette Galas, Hannah Walinska, Lillian Baer, Carol Lyn Conragan, Ann Gifford, Penny Warfield, Kathy Walters, Wendy Klee, Carol Braunshausen, and Varda Nowack-Goldstein.

A special thanks is due to Jill and John Freidenrich and Helen and Peter Bing, for their generous support of this book. Jill is the cofounder of the Community Breast Health Project in Palo Alto, California, and has been an inspiration to me. To

Karen Nierenberg, executive director, and Amy Moody, program director, of the Community Breast Health Project, thank you for your willingness to listen to my ideas and support the pilot program in 2001. The program has flourished in the warmth of the small living room at CBHP since its inception.

Eight of my friends and colleagues were willing to receive the book in its earliest form, rough and raw, and give me their reactions and encouragement. Thank you to my husband, John Renner, and to Jill Freidenrich, Lynn Rhodes, Gingie Halloran, Karen Jandorf, Chapin Day, Daphne Slocombe, and Molly Polidoroff, for knowing how to help me improve my draft, yet offer sincere encouragement that a writer truly needs to see a project like this through to completion. Thank you to Ellen Shuck for being so willing to proofread the pages. And special thanks to my daughters, Elinor and Claire, because they are always great cheerleaders for their mother.

Thank you to Pat Schneider, founder of Amherst Writers & Artists, and my editor. Pat believed in the book, and she has believed in me. I am deeply indebted to Pat and to Peter for their tender care, time and support of this book project.

Thank you also to Barbara Werden for her insightful guidance in book design and publishing, and finally, to Amherst Writers & Artists Press for making it possible to tell the story of our healing journey to a wider audience.

SHARON BRAY

A Healing Journey

Introduction

THE CALL TO WRITING

vocation *n.* a calling, from vocāre, to call.
The Barnhart Concise Dictionary of Etymology

I have always loved to write, and I had always wanted to be a writer. After many failed attempts to take action and realize my dreams, I registered, in the spring of 2000, for a weeklong creative writing workshop that was scheduled for the Graduate Theological Union's summer session in Berkeley, California. By August, when the workshop actually began, my life had changed dramatically. Soul weary from my life as CEO of a dying nonprofit, I had been diagnosed with an early-stage breast cancer and just completed seven weeks of radiation therapy. I had resigned from my job and taken a consulting assignment as the interim executive director for a Palo Alto–based nonprofit organization, The Community Breast Health Project. CBHP was founded in 1993 by Jill Freidenrich, a breast cancer survivor, and her surgeon, Dr. Ellen Mahoney, with the mission of improving the lives of people touched by breast cancer. Today, CBHP serves as an educational resource and a community center for all who are concerned about breast cancer and breast health, and provides support groups, information, and outreach into the larger community.

Who can say what forces were driving the coalescence of events that summer leading me to the proposal and pilot for the first writing group of breast cancer survivors? Some might call it serendipity or planned happenstance, but just a few months after my workshop experience in Berkeley, my own journey through cancer and healing became the impetus to develop a writing group program for women whose lives had been affected by a diagnosis of cancer.

This little book tells the story of my journey to become a writing group leader for women living with cancer. It is a story of a courageous group of women writing through their experiences of cancer, and it is the story of their journey through cancer and into healing. Healing, in the context of cancer, takes many forms. Writing does not cure cancer, but it helps to heal the wounded spirit. It helps us come to terms with our illnesses and our lives. It helps us to find community and support with each other.

This is the story of our experience of writing together and the power of writing to heal. The book is intended for those of you whose lives have been touched by cancer, for those of you who have felt the pain of having someone close to you diagnosed with cancer, for those of you who write as a way to make sense out of your lives, and for those of you who want to lead writing groups, whether for cancer survivors or any group of individuals who are dealing with life traumas and hardships. This is the story of the journey of women writing together through cancer.

August 2000. At the time I began the workshop in Berkeley, I had no idea how my life would change. After an exhilarating week writing with Pat Schneider, the founder of Amherst Writers & Artists, I returned to my daily routine and work. Yet the excitement of what I had experienced lingered on. Something ignited deep within me, and I talked enthusiastically to anyone who would listen about my experience in Pat's workshop. I enrolled for a number of other writing workshops at local universities and read book after book on creative writing. One morning, the development director at Community Breast Health Project (CBHP) placed an article from *MAMM Magazine* on my desk. Entitled "Scribbling My Way to Spiritual Well-Being," the author, Musa Mayer, described her experience with the healing power of writing, and in it she referred to the work of James Pennebaker, a psychologist at the University of Texas in Austin, whose research had shown that emotional—and in some cases, physical—healing is helped by writing. The article described my own experience with writing. I read it with keen interest, and before I knew it, the sparks of an idea were kindled into flame. I searched eagerly on the Internet and in the library for more articles and research and quickly found Pennebaker's book, *Opening Up: The Healing Power of Expressing Emotions.* I was hooked.

Pennebaker's research struck a responsive chord. Writing had always been an important part of my own personal healing. My shelves are filled with journals full of thoughts and feelings—poetry and prose that are evidence of my life. I always used writing in my professional practice, incorporating reflective writing exercises with the individuals I counseled during career transition. In teaching my graduate career counseling classes at Santa Clara University, I incorporated the use of learning journals as an integral part of the courses, encouraging my students to integrate their career and life stories into existing adult learning and career development theory.

Now I was intrigued by the growing body of research that supported the power of writing, not only to enable creative self-expression and self-insight but its power to heal the human spirit. Could I find a way to involve myself more deeply in this work? Suddenly, the seeds of my new vocation were sown. I knew that a return to full-time management roles was no longer something I could consider. Within months, I began leading my first writing group for women diagnosed with breast cancer. Later, I expanded my work to include groups of at-risk teenage girls, bereaved adults, senior citizens, and any adults who simply wanted to write in a safe and supportive environment.

From the inception of the first breast cancer writing group, I witnessed an exhilarating unfolding of the power of writing to enable self-discovery, creativity, self-reflection, healing, community, and ultimately, one's own spirituality: connection to self, others, and the world. Since my first intensive workshop experience with Pat Schneider in the summer of 2000, I have continued to deepen my own writing practice and lead writing groups for women living with cancer. It is powerful, affirming work, and the women who write the stories of their journey through cancer are an inspiration. It is my privilege to lead these groups, to write with the women, and to learn from our shared experience. In the pages that follow, I invite you to experience our journey of writing and healing, to be touched by the women's stories, to learn from our experience, and to explore the extraordinary power of writing together through cancer.

Pedestal

By Hanna Walinska

Symmetry is gone
Painfully
The old goddess has fallen
The old goddess is dead.

Discard the old image
Oh fateful
Because our new lady is truly great
To us all.

She is a wounded warrior
Give her time to lick her wounds
Oh fateful
Because our new lad is as fierce
As a gladiator.

Asymmetric is our new lady
But she is seeking balance
Trust me
Oh fateful
This one will not fall too easily
Though she knows
She may die soon.

I

Creating a Healing Environment

I now see pain, loss and grief as the basis for virtually every act of cultural creation.
LOUISE DESALVO

Breast cancer is primarily a woman's disease, and not surprisingly, many women have written about their experiences with it. Many of the books on the subject are oriented toward self-help or memoir. Other authors, like Audrey Lorde, Lucille Clifton, and Marilyn Hacker, have written stunning prose or poetry out of their cancer journey. When I tried to find books about writing approaches used to deal with the emotional impact of a cancer diagnosis, I found several, but they were predominantly oriented toward personal journaling. Few, if any, went beyond solitary self-expression; none that I could find discussed how to establish a supportive writing community for individuals suffering from cancer or other life traumas. Yet each book had its value in demonstrating the therapeutic benefit of writing through the experience of cancer or other life traumas, and in the absence of a writing group experience, the tools and tips for personal journaling I read in several books were invaluable.

Pat Schneider's first book on writing, *The Writer as An Artist*, described the pioneering writing method of Amherst Writers & Artists, focusing on creating a nurturing environment for the wounded writer to experience the safety to come out into the open, be healed, and flourish. I searched for the book prior to taking her workshop, but discovered it had gone out of print. Pat recently revised her original work and wrote a new book, *Writing Alone and with Others,* which is an excellent resource for any writer or workshop leader.

But I left for the Graduate Theological Union and my first creative writing workshop with Pat Schneider knowing little about the Amherst Writers & Artists method, except that it had been successfully used in a wide variety of groups where the power of a shared writing experience was evident. One only has to view the award-winning documentary *Tell Me Something I Can't Forget,* which featured Pat's work with low-income women in a Chicopee, Massachusetts, housing project to be convinced of extraordinary potential in helping women find their voices by writing together and telling their stories. I would soon come to know the AWA method intimately and experience its applicability and power firsthand as I began leading my writing groups for women living with cancer.

Like any new writers, the women in my breast cancer groups came to the first workshop with a mixture of excitement and apprehension. Their early experiences with writing had oftentimes been hurtful. "At first I think I was very apprehensive," Judy told me. "Every other experience I had with writing involved lots of red ink and questionable remarks across the pages. I never had anything but unenthusiastic criticism connected with the writing experience."

Creating the Safety to Write

Not only is it important to create a safe and supportive writing environment for the creative process to flourish, but such an environment also enables our writing to truly be healing. Providing a safe and non-judgmental space for individuals' writing voices and creativity to emerge, and defining an approach that protects that safety were the most important aspects of my training with Amherst Writers & Artists. Recognizing the wounded writer in all of us, Schneider created a methodology and a writing environment in the context of her workshops that, while taking seriously writing as an art form, also invited that wounded self into the open, to be affirmed and loved unconditionally, to heal and flourish. Isn't this at the heart of art? Of helping professions? Of ministering to another? Of healing?

Pat Schneider fostered an extraordinary movement in her AWA workshops. I have taken many other writing workshops, and I have experienced some similarities in approaches, but none was as clear or distinct as the AWA method in informing my initial work with the cancer writing groups. At the heart of the AWA method are clear-cut and simple guidelines. These are outlined and beautifully documented in Pat Schneider's new book, *Writing Alone and with Others,* published by Oxford University Press, a must-have for any writing group leader. The following is excerpted from *Writing Alone and with Others,* with permission by Pat Schneider and Oxford University Press:

The Amherst Writers & Artists Workshop Method

THE FIVE ESSENTIAL AFFIRMATIONS:

1. Everyone has a strong, unique voice.
2. Everyone is born with creative genius.
3. Writing as an art form belongs to all people, regardless of economic class or educational level.
4. The teaching of craft can be done without damage to a writer's original voice or artistic self-esteem.
5. A writer is someone who writes.

TWELVE BASIC PRINCIPLES FOR A HEALTHY WORKSHOP:

1. Write together in workshop and invite, but do not pressure, members to read what they have just written.
2. Do not allow the workshop to critique or correct first-draft

work that has just been written in the workshop.

3. Allow great diversity in age, experience, style, and genre in your workshop.

4. Assume all written work to be fictional unless the writer volunteers that it is autobiographical.

5. Encourage workshop members to be honest with both praise and critical suggestion in responding to work in manuscript form. Be rigorous and honest in your own responses.

6. Give your workshop a wide variety of exercises.

7. Write along with your workshop members, read that work aloud, and invite response.

8. If one person is making the group unworkable, ask that person to leave.

9. Do not be thrown off-center by anyone else's expertise; be realistic and without defensiveness about your own limitations and strengths as leader.

10. Stress confidentiality.

11. Help people try out new forms in writing.

12. In moments of genuine crisis, be ready to abandon all "practices"; follow your own instinct.

In the first weeks that I led the pilot program at the Community Breast Health Project, I watched and listened in awe as each woman opened up and began to write deeply and beautifully. I saw us cry together; I heard us laugh together. I saw the power of writing together to heal our wounded spirits, and I was hungry to learn more about the therapeutic benefits of writing, especially writing together during the diagnosis and treatment of cancer. I began searching the bookstores and library shelves for anything I could find that dealt with the personal experience of cancer.

Writing & Therapy

Simply speaking the truth heals.
RACHEL NAOMI REMEN

There is little doubt that writing together has therapeutic benefits, but a writing group is not a therapy group. Nowhere has the need to understand the differences between the two been more evident than in the writing groups I lead for women living with breast cancer. At CBHP, where I began my first groups, a number of therapist-led support groups are offered for women with breast cancer. Although the women who attended my writing group came to write, they began to describe the group as their primary cancer support group, so powerful was the experience of writing together. How then are the cancer writing groups similar to other cancer support groups?

The shared experience of cancer defines our writing group in a unique way. Not only do the women come because they want to write, they come because they also want to use writing to help them deal with the realities of cancer and their emotions in response to it. How we go about creating a safe and supportive environment for writing together has a lot in common with creating a safe and supportive therapy group for breast cancer survivors. Yet it is critical to understand the distinctions between the two, for the temptation in leading a healing writing workshop may be to cross that delicate boundary between writing that is therapeutic and writing as a therapeutic intervention.

An AWA-method writing group for breast cancer survivors should be, first and foremost, a group focused on writing: writing creatively about one's life and one's cancer journey. The only requirement for joining is that the women are survivors of or living with breast cancer—or other cancer. Several times women came to the group with cancers other than breast cancer, discovering the flyer in a hospital waiting room or hearing about the groups from friends and colleagues. "Do you take women with any cancer?" they called and asked. My response was an immediate "Yes." No woman with any kind of cancer has ever been turned away.

Dr. David Spiegel, professor of psychiatry at Stanford University in California, has explored different therapeutic treatment models and their impact on metastatic cancer patients. He has focused primarily on the supportive-expressive group treatment model based on building social bonds to encourage discussion of common problems among cancer patients.

Breast cancer can have a profound effect on self-image. The shock of diagnosis, followed by a whirlwind of decision making, treatment, and the adjustment to a radically altered body, leaves us with little opportunity to come to terms with a changed sense of self. Having cancer, Spiegel observes, "is like being shot by a sniper."

When I invited the women in my writing group to talk about their cancer experience, they described the shock of their own diagnoses. "I experienced cancer through my sister's journey first, her lumpectomy and mastectomy," Karen wrote. "She was five years younger than me. I thought I had escaped . . . but after dinner one night, I touched my breast and found a lump. I knew it was a tumor. The bottom fell out of my life."

The diagnosis of breast cancer—or any cancer—creates, as Karen has described, an extraordinary loss of self. Everything we have taken for granted about ourselves is blown asunder. Grieving for that lost or altered self is a necessary part of coming to terms with cancer in our lives.

Loneliness also accompanies the diagnosis of cancer. Spiegel observed that social isolation is a frequent complaint. Cancer undoes us. We suddenly find ourselves in a world teeming with confusion and uncertainty. Time and time again, the women in my writing groups have told me that they have often felt more comfort and understanding from other women who have shared the experience of cancer than they do from friends and family. Jean said of the women in the writing group, "I feel supported and loved by them. I can offer them kindness and support too. There is healing in giving as well as receiving."

Yet the demands of cancer and its treatment take up time, ironically decreasing opportunities for interactive social support that is so needed. Irena described the emotional journey of her cancer as "very mixed. I lost friends and gained friends. It was quite a test."

Spiegel's supportive-expressive therapy groups for cancer patients encourage emotional expression rather than trying to channel or suppress it. In these groups, emotion becomes a valued source of closeness rather than a cause of isolation. His research with metastatic cancer patients in supportive-expressive therapy groups demonstrated the power of social support to improve not only coping skills, but quality of life and even, in some cases, survival rates for metastatic breast cancer patients.

Allowing our fears out into the open also promotes the bonds of community. When we are safe enough to express to others our fears of death and dying, we also detoxify their power. Bringing our fears to the surface and telling them to one another makes them more manageable and less overwhelming. When we write together, all we may need is a nudge from a writing prompt and the safety to read aloud. When we help cancer patients face their fears directly, we create intimacy, what Spiegel refers to as "social glue."

Recently, one of our group members died from metastatic cancer, but until her body and her eyesight began to fail her completely, she faithfully attended each Wednesday's writing session. The support and community she felt with the women was deeply important to her. Just before her death, as she lay in a coma, I spoke with her daughter, who tearfully thanked me for creating the writing experience for breast cancer survivors. "The writing group," she said, "kept my mother going all these many weeks."

A social community that is safe and supportive can also improve our ability to cope with our illness. When we write and share our cancer journeys, we can hear how others have coped successfully with the disease; we can offer support and inspiration to one another. The poet Audrey Lorde knew this well, and her book *The Cancer Journals* is a powerful testimony to the importance of her writing and a supportive community in helping her face cancer. She wrote, "My work and the love of women kept me alive this past year. They are inseparable from each other. In the recognition of the existence of love lies the answer to despair. Work is that recognition given voice and name."

"Writing allows experience to take shape," Irena told me as she reflected on being part of the group. "A lot has opened up, and it is possible to start to make peace with it."

Jean agreed, saying that the writing exercises have helped her to bring her feelings to the surface and to let go of her cancer experience as a negative one.

Varda found writing enabled her to be "more accepting of myself. . . . I have come to think of my cancer experience as more positive than negative."

Dr. Michael Lerner, cofounder of the Commonweal Cancer Help Program in Bolinas, California, said, "At the emotional level of healing, expressing the feeling gives you an opportunity to look at it. You've put it out there in a safe and supportive context, and now you can look at it. And as you look, the experience of the feeling begins to turn, and you begin to be able to step back from it, and to experience that you have a self separate from this terror or anxiety."

The act of writing forces us to externalize our experiences, and in writing together and reading aloud to a supportive audience, we begin to make sense of our lives, name our fears, and reframe our experience. Reframing experience is sense-making, and it allows us to learn and gain perspective. Dr. Rachel Naomi Remen, cofounder of Commonweal, described healing as "different from curing . . . Healing is . . . very close to the process of education."

"Cancer," Irena said quietly to me as we talked about the writing group experience, "has been a great teacher to me."

Honoring the Boundaries Between Therapy & Writing

Whenever I get somewhere, a poet has been there first.
SIGMUND FREUD

Art, Pat Schneider has asserted, is essential to every one of us. Each of us is a creator. Art has to be free to go wherever it needs to go, and pain often makes itself known first. Healing is often a by-product of artistic self-expression.

Sigmund Freud believed our creative imagination was instrumental in emotional healing, enabling us to relive and re-create experience in a symbolic way. This is the power of art. It gives expression to the originality in each of us. Our wounded emotions become the raw material for the creation of books, poems, plays, and symphonies. In this way, artistic expression has enormous therapeutic value.

Liberating our creativity and artistry is one of the most important aspects of the power of writing to heal. In the AWA writing methodology I use with my cancer groups, the distinction between art and therapy is clear. A writing group is not a therapy group. It is a writing group, concerned with liberating the artist in the person; yet, writing together can be very therapeutic.

Writing does have many benefits in common with some forms of therapy. Psychologist James Pennebaker, whose research explores the healing benefits of writing, has demonstrated clear parallels between the benefits of writing and therapy:

- Both can improve physical and psychological health.
- Both encourage self-reflection and greater insight.
- Both promote understanding and acknowledge emotions.

When I asked the women in our cancer group to comment on the most healing aspects of writing together, Judy responded, "The writing workshops have enabled me to feel good about myself during a time when chemo brain was raging rampantly, and my body was under massive assault. I have been allowed to rage at cancer, cry over losses, triumph at small steps accomplished. Thank you with all my heart."

Marcia said, "When I started the class, almost every writing assignment was a tearful one for me. After about nine months, I had worked through a lot of those raw, bottled emotions and now can write with more humor and, hopefully, wisdom."

Karen added, "It has all been wonderful and full of meaning, but the combination of writing in a group as friendships grow, forming bonds, sharing sorrows and laughter, has been invaluable."

In *Writing and Healing*, published by the National Council of Teachers of English, coauthor Marian MacCurdy notes that our knowledge of the writing process demands that writing instructors engage with the psyches of those we teach. Because of that, she believes that it is increasingly important for writing instructors to learn more about the process of therapy and its intersection with writing instruction, so that we can keep the lines between writing and therapy clear. One of the aspects of the AWA method that I have come to appreciate most as I lead my cancer groups is that the role of the leader is clearly defined. The leader creates and protects the facilitating environment that ensures the safety to write from our deepest selves.

For example, in the AWA method, all writing is assumed to be fiction, unless the writer needs to have it treated as autobiography. With the breast cancer group, it is very important to assume fiction, even though, again, 9.9 times out of 10, what emerges is the writer's own life experience. Treating it as fiction creates safety, neither allowing for others' interpretations of how the writer must have felt, nor the projection of our own experience onto the writer's. It also honors the way that our memory "fictionalizes" actual facts and remembers only the truth of the emotional experience; thus, assuming fiction makes it safe to write openly, honestly, and creatively. Marcia talked about how the AWA method supported her writing: "Establishing a safe environment and making only affirming comments really enables people to open up their deeper feelings. The affirmation and shared emotions build a swift intimacy that makes it acceptable to reveal anything."

The essential practices that are fundamental to the AWA method make it powerful as a "healing" methodology. The method of group leadership encourages the healing of our wounds as writers, and heals our traumas and our painful life experiences. We use the senses to evoke memory and imagery, while providing safety, confidentiality, and support to others by offering affirmations specific to the writer's language and imagery.

It is hardly a surprise that much more than the pain of cancer is written about in a breast cancer survivors' writing group. On any given evening, memories of childhood suffering, loneliness, alcoholic parents, or even abuse will make their way into the writing as readily as the dear and loving memories of our lives. Writing creates for us a watershed, a release, an opening up of our deepest humanity, and when we write from our deepest place and read it aloud, audible sighs and sounds of letting go can be heard around the room as the women listen to one another. They acknowledge and affirm the truth of one another's experience. Besides, as Rachel Remen stated, "Simply speaking the truth heals."

How I Write

By Neli Stascausky

I write without organizing rhythm or rhyme
in my mind
Like pure water from a spring
into a crystal bowl
the words flow from my heart to my hand.

I let the sunlight give them life and then
gently, move them to feel the spark,
All natural, unstructured, not judged.

I feel free at last! And my words
dance in someone's mind
to their own rhythm and rhyme
and I'm alive!

2

When Writing Is Healing

WHAT THE RESEARCH TELLS US

I have woven a parachute out of everything
broken. My scars are my shield.
WILLIAM STAFFORD

The literature on the subject of healing and writing is
expanding rapidly as we embrace more holistic, artistic, and
spiritual aspects of emotional and physical healing. I discovered a vast array of exploration and research in psychology,
healthcare, literature, and writing. My intent in this chapter is
to highlight some of the research I found most informative
and supportive of my experience and observations of writing
together through cancer.

The connection between writing and healing is not new.
For many years, poets and novelists have used their writing to
transform trauma and heal themselves. Suzette Henke, author
of *Shattered Subjects*, suggests that traumatic experiences of
poets and writers are common to those suffered by ordinary
people in the course of modern life. Scriptotherapy, a broad
term that refers to the use of books, plays, and poetry to help
people solve problems, involves the deliberate use of writing
to heal. Scriptotherapy offers a psychological sanctuary for
writers "in which to reconstruct ourselves after shattering
experiences," Henke writes. She cites many examples, many as

early as the late nineteenth century, including Virginia Woolf, writing through the repercussions of her own trauma, and Anais Nin, describing her own writing as an "antitoxin" to despair. Writing, whether in poetry or prose, allows us to say the unsayable, opening up our buried pain and emotions, and to heal.

Linda McCarriston, a contemporary poet, wrote an award-winning book of poetry, *Eva-Mary,* her experience of domestic violence growing up in a working-class family. "I felt driven to attempt to write poems from these very difficult experiences of my childhood," she said. Her poetry allowed her to find expression, validation, and truth to build her life.

"Stories are antibodies against illness and pain," Anatole Broyard wrote as he examined his own illness. Writing in his book, *Intoxicated by My Illness,* he stated, "always in emergencies we invent narratives. We describe what is happening, as if to confine the catastrophe." Part of the healing power in writing is that it gives us a way to maintain control over our lives and move beyond thinking of ourselves as victims in the face of traumatic experiences.

Writing gets our feelings in the open, and emotional expression is an important aspect of healing from upsetting life events. When we bury our emotions, we are also blocking our ability to recover from illness or trauma. Repressed emotions are counterproductive to healing. If we silence our stories, Louise DeSalvo wrote in her book, *Writing As a Way of Healing,* it can adversely affect our health. Writing allows us to get emotions out into the open and onto the page, where we can truly "see" what we are feeling. Opening up and telling our stories appear to unleash our body's potential to heal.

However, despite a long history of writers using their own writing to heal from grief and trauma, psychologists have only relatively recently begun to amass a body of empirical research that investigates the conditions under which writing can be healing. The results have been impressive, and, according to some researchers, writing may be our single most effective therapeutic tool for healing.

Opening Up: The Work of James Pennebaker

James Pennebaker is the acknowledged pioneer in the psychological research examining the healing benefits of writing. In a number of instances, his studies have consistently shown that writing can positively affect people's lives and health. Writing, he has concluded, allows us to confront traumas and put them to rest. It allows us to heal.

Ann, one of the women in my original pilot, said, "The writing was healing in letting me see how I felt. I could look at the writing and see a part of myself on the paper."

Jean agreed, "I have been able to explore my issues more deeply: issues that exist because of cancer and issues that result from other life experiences. . . . I am able to use the writing to stop my mind from fretting over the fact of cancer and treatment."

Pennebaker's research is a must-read for any aspiring workshop leader who wishes to understand the research that demonstrates why writing can be healing. *Opening Up: The Healing Power of Expressing Emotions,* first published in 1990 and revised in 1997, summarizes much of his original research. Among the many findings, Pennebaker and his colleagues found that the benefits of writing are consistent across a broad range of different populations, including all economic levels and racial/ethnic groups. In certain conditions, writing can have positive impact on immune functioning, and it has also been associated with lower levels of depression as well as reduced pain and use of medication. Why, then, is writing such a powerful tool for healing?

The Conditions for Writing to Be Healing

Pennebaker's studies indicated that certain conditions must be present for writing to be truly healing. As I have led my cancer writing groups, I have found that the essential practices of the Amherst Writers & Artists method naturally create these healing conditions. Both stress confidentiality; there are no corrections or criticism; individuals experience a free-write of emotions and thoughts in a regular timed routine; and above all, they experience safety in which to write freely. The four necessary conditions for writing to be healing are:

Emotional processing

People must be given the freedom to invoke their feelings—positive and negative—when writing about an emotional topic. Writing in a safe and supportive environment, where feedback focuses only on the specific and positive aspects of one's writing, enables the freedom for honest emotional expression. The writing prompts have no conditions; they simply evoke images, memories, whatever is there to write, and in the timed writing the writer will go deeper quickly. Anything goes. Anything is allowed in one's writing.

A coherent story

The greatest health benefits occur when people write a "coherent" story—one that involves structure, causal explanation, repetition of themes, awareness and appreciation of a listener's perspective. During the timed writing exercises I use in our cancer groups, what often emerges may be only the beginning of a story, an incident that opens into the heart of a much larger story. Over the several weeks we write together, it is expanded and deepened and becomes complete. We all have a natural tendency to create story, whether in the form of a poem or a personal narrative, and the use of a variety of writing prompts opens up the memories so critical to story formation. Another important element in the AWA method supports the creation of story: the expectation of reading aloud, which also foists the presence of an audience into the writing experience. To keep our listeners with us, we implicitly create what is natural among humans: story.

Postwriting processing

After writing, people continue to think about their writing; it lingers in their minds for days afterward. Those of us who write together each evening leave with the stories and poems written in the moment, in response to writing prompts. Often, the women will tell me that, in the days that follow, they continue to think about and expand the writing that began in the group session. I cannot even count the times that the women have returned to the following session, telling me, "I couldn't stop thinking about it . . . ," or "I kept working on that piece I started in class. . . ." Often, we go home and continue to write, develop, and expand what was begun in the workshop. "It makes me think," Clarissa said to me. "Even after the workshops, I keep thinking. I am getting my vitality back and ideas for paintings and prints. Writing gets our feelings and experiences outside of ourselves, available for viewing, and in this way, helps to promote self-understanding and perspective."

A trustworthy setting

The safety and confidentiality of the setting in which writing occurs must be protected in order for people to write true. Providing the safety and supportive environment in which the women can find their voices is at the core of the AWA methodology. The basic practices and presence of a supportive leader are instrumental to ensuring that safety—trustworthiness—is preserved for every writer. Creativity, as well as the ability to write openly and honestly, needs safety.

A fundamental practice of the AWA workshop method is to have the leader write with the group—as honestly and deeply as everyone else. This aspect is critical to creating the safety that is so necessary in writing together. I write and read my writing aloud as I invite participants to do, sometimes surprised by the forgotten memories that spring forth onto my page or the accompanying rush of emotion. One night, as I perused the array of objects I'd placed on the table as prompts, I picked up a police evidence bag and sat down to write, not knowing where my writing would take me. Earlier that week, my mother had been admitted to hospice care after a long, slow deterioration from Alzheimer's disease.

Evidence. It's not enough that she wears diapers now, incontinent and oblivious to her bodily functions. They want evidence.

Never mind that she can't walk anymore. My mother used to walk six or eight miles a day. Now she sits in a wheelchair with vacant eyes; her head nods into her lap. Sometimes she can't even get out of bed. But they want evidence.

"Hey Mom. It's me, Sharon. Remember?" Her eyes are cloudy, a thick mental fog surrounds her brain. She descends further into the darkness, gone from me. She cannot form a sentence; her words turn to gibberish. She tries to lift the spoon to her lips, a woman-child struggling to remember how to eat. But still they want evidence. Evidence she will die soon. Evidence she will not live beyond six months. Evidence.

When Writing Is Healing

According to Pennebaker and his colleagues, writing that is healing also has a number of key attributes, which are summarized briefly in the following paragraphs.

Translating trauma into language

In order to have health gains, a traumatic or disturbing event needs to be translated into language. When we convert emotions and images into words, it changes the way we think, organize, and react emotionally to the traumatic event. When we integrate our thoughts and feelings, we can more easily construct a coherent narrative of the experience, one that allows us to reflect and gain insight.

In Pennebaker's studies, people reported feeling better for several weeks following the research task of writing about emotionally upsetting events. The researchers discovered that when people write about trauma, the changes they experience are similar to those they experience when talking to a therapist. "I cannot imagine my life without this group," one writer told me. "It helped me so much in getting through it [the cancer experience]."

Encouraging the exploration of emotions

No single writing topic produced greater health benefits than another. The researchers discovered the most important aspect of introducing a writing topic was to encourage people to explore their emotions and thoughts, no matter what the content.

Time and time again, as the women in my cancer groups read what they have written, their voices break or their eyes well up with tears. I often hear comments like "I didn't know I was going there . . ." or "I didn't know I still felt so strongly." As they read aloud, perhaps they truly hear themselves as never before. The writing exercises I use in my cancer writing groups act as latchkeys, opening up the storehouse of memories and the emotions associated with them. I have observed that nearly any prompt will take us to whatever emotions and life events are waiting to be expressed. "Trust the process," I remember Pat Schneider saying in my first workshop with her. "The writing will take you to wherever you need to go." The process of writing and reading aloud in a safe and supportive environment seems to be more important than any particular prompt or topic.

The importance of emotional expression in healing has been validated and expanded by many other researchers, including some studies conducted specifically with women diagnosed with breast cancer, such as those by David Spiegel, Annette Stanton, and Sharon Danoff-Burg.

Stanton and Danoff-Burg highlighted the importance of expressive disclosure in the adjustment process for women diagnosed with cancer. They investigated the impact of emotional processing on women's adjustment to the disease, defining emotional processing as "active, intentional attempts to acknowledge, explore meanings, and come to an understanding of one's emotions and emotional expression." In such expression of emotions, a woman may become better able to distinguish between what she can and cannot control in her experience of cancer and her life.

David Spiegel's supportive-expressive group therapy work with metastatic breast cancer patients, described in an earlier section in this book, also stresses the importance of emotional expression in healing. One of Spiegel's major findings was that women in his intervention group, those who experienced the supportive-expressive group therapy process after treatment, lived about twice as long as the women in the control group, who received no group therapy.

Stanton and Danoff-Burg also found that writing had healing benefits for the women who were suffering from breast cancer. Despite its sometimes painful task, writing helped the women to think about their cancer experience, clarifying where their life was and where they wanted it to go. For writing to be beneficial, Stanton and Danoff-Burg discovered, it was not necessary to address painful thoughts and feelings head on. Rather, simply writing about the cancer experience—opening it up and expressing one's feelings and thoughts—had positive benefits for the women.

Overcoming isolation

When we are diagnosed with breast cancer, it is frightening and deeply upsetting. We can feel stigmatized or alienated from family or friends, loved ones who mean well but cannot share in our fears and experience. "I felt alone," one woman told me, "although my friends and family were wonderful." Women struggle to come to terms with losing one or both breasts during surgery or, in chemotherapy, the loss of hair and other bodily distortions. It is easy to feel stigmatized by the nature of the illness and its treatment. Writing can help overcome the isolation. Pennebaker's research revealed that, in certain "stigmatized" groups, writing improved the level of collective self-esteem that individuals experienced.

In our writing group, the shared journey of cancer united the women in a unique way. Writing together bonded and strengthened the positive self-regard the women had for themselves and for each other. "Writing together has given me confidence," Karen said. "I feel I can be seen. I feel less alone."

Writing together about our cancer experience helps to heal our damaged self-esteem as it builds a sense of shared understanding. Writing gives us back our voices, voices that are sometimes lost when we suffer a life-threatening illness like cancer or bodily disfigurement from treatment. Judy was grateful for the writing group experience in helping her feel understood and supported. "I have been able to explore and share my hidden terrors, my hopes and joys with this compassionate group of women," she wrote. "I've been able to explore my feelings within the warm and welcoming embrace of those who are making the same passage."

Writing in the presence of others

The importance of writing in the presence of other people, showing that writing or speaking about one's experiences in the presence of someone else, even if that person is not a therapist, helps people to heal from painful life events. Judy attributes much of the healing power of her writing experience to the act of sharing her cancer story in a supportive group of women. "Writing together provides a supportive environment that is . . . important to my healing process. Sharing our experiences with this life-threatening illness has changed us. It is marvelous."

A balanced narrative

A balanced narrative, one that includes both positive and negative emotion words as well as reflective and causal words, indicated better health improvement in Pennebaker's studies. While I do not monitor or track specific progress, it is interesting to observe how, over the many weeks we write together, the women begin to gain strength and confidence, and their writing shifts from being predominantly those full of raw or angry emotions directed at their cancer diagnosis to becoming more hopeful and inclusive of their whole lives. As our writing becomes healing, the painful negative emotions give way to questioning, acceptance, and resolution, or at the very least, those are considered with an eye to understanding and self-insight.

Constructing a story

Perhaps it is because of the deep tradition of storytelling in human evolution, but out of all of Pennebaker's findings, I was most intrigued by this: most associated with healing writing is the construction of story. Pennebaker found that merely having a story was not enough. It was critical to create a coherent narrative out of it, one that could help to organize the emotional effects of an experience as well as the experience itself. In the cancer writing groups, no matter the prompt, the women would naturally shape their thoughts, feelings, and memories into story or, perhaps, narrative poetry.

Writing together and reading aloud promote story creation, which may be what makes the activity potentially more healing than solitary writing or journaling through illness or trauma. The qualities that make a good oral tale, a moving memoir, or a compelling piece of fiction are also those that make a coherent story, something researchers have discovered as critical to writing that is healing. When we are writing and reading aloud together, we are more aware of the audience and our listeners than if we are journaling for ourselves. The writing exercises I introduce each evening provide the trigger to emotions, thoughts, and images, but the act of writing and reading aloud in the presence of others facilitates the creation of stories.

For writing to be truly healing, as far as the psychological research is concerned, it is critical for us to confront our anxieties and problems by creating a story to explain and understand our pasts and our current life concerns. It doesn't matter so much what kind of story we create, whether an autobiography or a fictional narrative. The more detailed, organized, vivid, and lucid our writing becomes, the greater the benefits we derive from it. And the more that writing succeeds in being descriptive, lucid, and vivid, the more engaging it is for the reader or the listener. Simply put, our human tradition of storytelling, or story construction, as a way to make sense of our worlds is what is most highly associated with healing, either mental or physical. Opening up, sharing our emotions and our life stories, helps to heal us and make us whole.

In *Writing As a Way of Healing*, Louise De Salvo wrote, "When we share our writing, someone else knows what we've been through. Someone else cares. Someone has heard our voice. Someone else understands. We learn that we are no longer alone and that we no longer need to be alone." Sometimes, it seems, we search for answers to life's problems when they have been there, as part of the fabric of our human existence, just within our reach, all of the time.

Dancing with Regret

By Varda Nowack Goldstein

Late in the night I dance with Regret, dipping and gliding through bad choices and unforgiven hurts. Through the ballroom window I see distant hills shrouded in the purple swirls of clouds tinted by fog. The shadowed light obscures my view of the horizon.

The tempo picks up as we glide past faint images of my parents waltzing in bare feet into the dawn, having carefully practiced each step and turn until they moved as one body. Even as I dance faster, I am aware of my growing fatigue. Regret whispers that some things are no longer possible. Again, my partner leans close to remind me of the time I should have spent as a sister and a mother, and that life is as illusionary as a soap bubble floating lightly by and then gone.

I find myself facing into a black-edged shadow as the music ends. Regret has slipped into the corner and asked my memories to speak. Standing alone, I hear my father as he faded from this world, "It all went so fast. . . . Life went so fast." My companion reminds me that those I loved are gone, and that I am dancing with a haunting and relentless suitor.

Before my illness, I viewed my life as a bright meadow rolling endlessly toward distant hills. Days and nights flowed past me without defined beginnings and endings. Although I aged, I still viewed my future as a meadow without fences.

When I awoke with cancer, Regret was my first visitor.

So today as the morning light rises, I breathe in the cold, clear air of the day, knowing full well that Regret will once again be my faithful evening companion.

3

From Campfires to Writing Groups

THE HEALING POWER OF STORY

> We need stories.... They are a fundamental unit
> of knowledge, the foundation of memory, essential
> to the way we make sense of our lives.
> BILL BUFORD

"All suffering is bearable," Isak Dinesen wrote, "if it is seen as part of a story." Story creation is as old as humankind's use of language. The rituals of gathering around campfires at night, telling stories and singing ballads, were deeply important to our ancient tribal ancestors. Through stories, we shared the events, values, and beliefs that defined us and shaped our communities. Story provided social glue. Storytelling was an interactive experience between teller or singer and listener. Story, some historians and psychologists believe, defined our humanity. Our ancient myths and legends explained the complexities of the world: creation, moral lessons, fire, lightning, or floods. In creating and telling our stories, our ancestors came to understand and make sense of their worlds, just as we use narratives to make sense of our lives today.

Each person's life is a story, and we are always discovering, through the finding and telling of our stories, who we are and what we are becoming. Stories help us understand how and why something has occurred and prepare us to deal with it.

Through story, we come together and share the experience of our lives. In creating and telling our stories, we discover our shared humanity.

When major or upsetting life events happen to us in the normal ebb and flow of our lives, they are often difficult for us to comprehend. If a marriage fails, a friend dies, our career derails, or, as with the women in my writing groups, we are diagnosed with breast cancer or another life-threatening disease, we can think of little else. We mull the event over and over, pummeling ourselves with questions, trying to understand and make sense of it. We feel deeply. Opening up the emotions that surround our traumas and losses by constructing story out of our experience helps us to heal. If we can't confront our feelings about an upsetting experience, they remain buried beneath the surface, making it difficult to gain perspective or resolve them. We find ourselves thinking, dreaming, and talking about the upsetting event for days, weeks, months, or even, as I once experienced in my own family, for years.

I was a senior in college when late one autumn night my parents' home caught fire and burned to the ground. The experience was highly traumatic for both my mother and father, and in the aftermath of the loss, my mother was consumed by a deep and consuming anguish, and she blamed my father for the tragedy. The fire remained an unresolved source of pain between them until my father's death over twenty-five years later. My mother continued the replay of the fire over and over in her mind; years later, she talked of the fire as if it had just happened, the blame as alive as it had been years before. Hers was a continuous replay of emotion that never became a balanced narrative or coherent story, one that could have helped her to heal her emotions and let go of her pain and anguish. Creating and telling our stories have the power to make us whole.

Stories Make Sense of Life

A single event like the diagnosis of cancer has very different meanings for different individuals, and a single writing exercise will yield as many different responses as there are writers in the group. The beauty of a narrative is that our individual uniqueness holds the universal truths we share with others. Anais Nin once said, "We write to taste life twice, in the moment, and in retrospection," and many writers have expressed the fact that we find the universal in the particular.

Once a complex event is put into a story format, Pennebaker concluded, it is simplified. We don't have to work as hard to figure it out or bring structure and meaning to it. Translating our distress into story allows us the perspective to forget or move beyond it. Writing our stories certainly gives us a chance to live life twice, but more importantly, it gives us an opportunity to make sense out of our lives, understand how we have changed or what we have learned from major life events. Healing is also learning, and the retrospective look that allows us to find the meaning in our life's experiences is key to reaping healing benefits from writing.

Translating the pain and struggle of cancer into insight and learning is a gradual process. The emotions attached to diagnosis, surgery, bodily distortions, and the aftermath of treatment are deep and complex. Writing about our cancer experiences and releasing the dam of difficult emotions surrounding them is the journey we travel together in the writing group. To heal, we not only need to write freely, but also the time to make sense of what we have written.

One of the women in my group shared a long, poignant piece of writing with me, in which she described her nightmare of misdiagnosis that resulted in the loss of both her breasts. "Is it publishable?" she asked. I read it carefully, moved time and again by her words, feeling tears or chills at the horror of her experience. But the narrative was still raw and bleeding, full of anger and self-recrimination. It lacked balance. I responded gently, suggesting that yes, she had a story that needed to be told to many women one day, but first, I hoped she would continue to simply let the experience pour out of her and onto the pages of her notebook. She was grateful and replied, "Thank you for taking such care with my writing." She acknowledged she still needed to heal before she turned it into a finished piece. She realized, once she brought her story into the open, that she still was too close to it, needing more time to heal from her experience and learn from it.

Sharing Story Builds Community

Hearing our words aloud in the presence of others is a powerful experience. Having an audience, whether readers or listeners, is an important aspect of fostering writing that is healing. Telling our stories to others requires the appreciation of the listener's perspective. We are also taken outside ourselves when we tell or read our stories to others, deepening our own understanding and perspective. Sharing our stories aloud with others may well open the doors to greater healing because it builds a strong and cohesive sense of community with others.

Regaining Control of Our Lives

Survivors, Anderson and MacCurdy contend, need to tell their stories in order to survive. Ann, one of the writers from the original pilot, told me that she felt she "was wounded in a number of ways by cancer, losing my positive feelings about my body and my health. I also lost a sense of control over my life."

Healing depends on our ability to gain control over what has engulfed us. In order to live our lives, we need to know and understand our buried truths. In the view of Anderson and MacCurdy, the major healing benefit of writing is in enabling us to recover and exert some measure of control over our pasts. Having some control in our lives helps us to weather difficult life events and to survive them. Writing, as so many of us have discovered, forces us to stop what we are doing and reflect on our lives. It is one of the few times we are free to see where we've been and where we're going without fear of recrimination or criticism. When we read aloud in the presence of a supportive audience who treat everything as "fiction" and respond only with what they liked or what was strong, the act of writing together can be enormously freeing. Healing can begin to occur.

When we re-create our life experiences through story, we can organize and remember events in a coherent fashion at the same time we integrate our thoughts and feelings. This is a key reason, according to Pennebaker, that stories help us to create a sense of predictability and control over our lives. When we give an upsetting experience structure and meaning, its emotional effects seem more manageable. We are less inclined to ruminate on a disturbing event, and gradually, our remembrances of painful experiences are diminished. We feel a sense of resolution.

Writing Alone or Writing Together

The safety and the privacy of a journal are important in making it a place where many of our demons, yearnings, and fears can first make their way into the open. I have kept a journal since childhood, and I cannot imagine my life without that precious time of writing in solitude. There are many resources, like those written by Deena Metzger and Kathleen Adams, that guide the prospective journal writer, and I have found them to be valuable in my own private writing.

Yet the solitary act of journaling, while beneficial in many ways, may sometimes result in rumination, a rewind and replay of the same negative tapes. Simply writing about negative events or venting our feelings doesn't necessarily produce the same health benefits as when story is created and shared in the presence of others. Karen, one of the writing group members, had tried journaling on her own as a way of confronting her cancer experience, but "I wasn't doing well at it," she said. "I journaled, but it was the prompts and the writing group that began to produce the changes in my writing and my feelings."

I have also turned to my journal in times of loss and life trauma. Dozens of notebooks line my bookshelves, testimony to the life I've lived. When my first marriage fell apart many years ago, and my husband accidentally drowned in the midst of our separation, I filled volumes of journals with my grief and rage. Years later, as I reread some of the passages, I discovered I had returned to the same painful questions over and over without moving forward from them. Only when, in my journal, I began to shape story in the form of poetry and memoir intended to be read by others did I begin to make sense of my experience and my emotions. Only then was I able to move on from those painful memories and extinguish their power.

Stories Shape Our Lives

Life stories occur everywhere: in our prose, poetry, letters, journals, songs, and folk tales. Some are silent; some are shared. Some are carried in artifacts or art. In recent years, along with the explosion of autobiographical and memoir writing, narrative psychology has gained momentum, its research aimed at understanding the ways in which stories shape our lives.

Practitioners of narrative psychology believe it is important for people to make sense of events in their lives by putting them into a storylike format. In narrative psychology, speaking our life stories, not unlike the process of reading aloud in our writing groups, involves the process of "telling with" another, and in doing so, discovering what our own life stories mean, naming the feelings associated with them, and discovering our own voices.

Reclaiming Our Own Stories

When we are diagnosed with cancer, we may sometimes lose our unique story and take on those of others. In a world of treatments, we are surrounded by physicians and medical expertise, and our own stories may be lost, something that has intrigued Rev. Steven Spidell, facilitator of a wellness class of healing stories at the University of Texas. "In the process of becoming patients," he said, "people often lose their stories. . . . With the chaos and disruption, they begin to tell the doctor's version of their story, the medical version, not their own. They get tunnel vision and forget who they were before. But people are fundamentally narrative based. They need to find meaning, make sense out of their disease."

Carolyn Schuk discovered her voice when, after a posttreatment examination, her physician offered reassurance and told her that she had an "excellent cosmetic result." Her wit overtook her as she described the exam during one of our writing sessions. In a piece entitled "Cruise Missiles, Big Israeli Breasts and Me," she told her own story. Here is the opening paragraph:

> Having recently undergone treatment for breast cancer, I think a lot about breasts these days. At the end of the treatment tunnel, grateful for the prospect of life and not having to make medical appointments, I listened to the doctor tell me I have "an excellent cosmetic result." I almost laughed in his face. Perhaps he thinks I'm going to start a new career as a stripper at 50. What he doesn't know is that I never thought I had a good cosmetic beginning, forget "result."

By the time Carolyn finished reading aloud, every woman in the room was nodding in understanding, smiling or laughing. Reclaiming our voices and our own stories is empowering. Shared laughter, as Norman Cousins so vividly demonstrated in his own recovery from critical illness, is also healing. By transforming our experiences into language, manipulating the words on the page, and articulating our emotional truths to others and ourselves, we become agents for our own healing. Bernadette, a staff member of CBHP who sometimes attended the writing group, said she was moved by the experience and being able to "witness how these women have opened their hearts, how they have changed through the sessions, and how they are starting to smile again at life."

"When you have a good cry," David Spiegel said of his therapeutic work with cancer patients, "you have a good laugh afterwards." It is hardly surprising that in recent years, there has been an explosion of personal writing and writing workshops, not only for their therapeutic benefits but also for the joy of self-expression.

"For our writing to be a healing experience," Louise DeSalvo writes, "we honor our pain, loss and grief." Writing transforms our deepest experiences into stories, poems, and prose, which bear witness to our lives. Writing is a work of art and bears testimony to our lives, our hurt and sorrow, and our courage and survival. It opens up our confusion and pain to understanding and the possibility of wholeness. It encourages us to take control of our lives. It gives us back our voices and our stories.

Women

By Bernadette Galas

Across the world, women
Across the age, women
Across the love, women
You are the stars of life
Across the time, women
You will shine forever
Across the age, women
You are the blossoms of love
Across the world, women
You are the tears and laughter
Across the suffering, women
You will never be alone
Across the life, women
You are soul and spirit
Women, women, women
Across my life, women
You are my sisters and friends
Thank you for being there.

4

Opening Up

THE FIRST EXPERIENCE IN AN AMHERST WRITERS & ARTISTS WORKSHOP

> Her voice belled forth, and the sunlight bent. I felt
> the ceiling arch, and knew that the nails up there
> took a new grip on whatever they touched. "I am
> your own way of looking at things," she said.
> "When you allow me to live with you, every
> glance at the world around you will be a sort of
> salvation." And I took her hand.
>
> WILLIAM STAFFORD, "When I Met My Muse"

"We are all artists." Pat Schneider was speaking to the group of us who had gathered for our first creative writing session at the Graduate Theological Seminary in Berkeley. "We are all writers." I wanted to believe her, but my internal critic pooh-poohed the notion. *We'll see,* I thought. *We'll see.*

I walked into Pat's creative writing workshop that summer, just weeks after being diagnosed with an early-stage breast cancer. I had soldiered my way, in a fog, through two lumpectomies and seven weeks of radiation. I had resigned my position as the CEO of a dying nonprofit in the midst of treatment, unable to stop its downward spiral. I was swinging on a trapeze somewhere between an overwhelming sense of professional failure and the realization that cancer was something happening to me. I was numb. Everything I had worked so hard to attain was unraveling. I turned inward and sought refuge in my journals. Journaling was a regular practice of mine begun many years before in a time of loss and upheaval. Writing had always been my refuge, but I never thought of myself as a writer even though I had written and published a few professional articles and a children's book several years earlier. To be called a writer, as far as I was concerned, was a privilege belonging to authors of best-selling novels or volumes of poetry, to editors and journalists writing for magazines and newspapers, or to those aspiring writers who were enrolled in academic MFA programs. "Writer" was not a title I bestowed upon myself. I simply wrote.

As I journaled, I filled page after page with endless questions and reexamined the events leading up to my diagnosis and resignation. Old hurts tumbled onto the page, and I replayed each one. I wrote in circles. I wrote backwards, looking for a clue, an answer: *why me?* I turned to writing poetry, but my internal critic trounced on every pallid attempt. I was blocked. One night in late May, I sat in my living room and cried into the telephone to my longtime friend Lynn Rhodes, a faculty member at the Graduate Theological Union's Pacific School of Religion. "Why don't you come to Berkeley and take Pat Schneider's workshop this summer?" She asked. "It's a week in July. You can stay at my house."

Now I sat quietly in a circle of men and women who wanted to write as badly as I did. I felt a wave of panic. What on earth was I doing here? We watched as Pat pulled a large bag to the middle of the floor and began laying out objects on a white cloth: a ring of ancient keys, a crucifix, a wooden spoon, a man's shaving brush, an empty whiskey bottle. She continued to reach inside the bag, pull out more objects—the "stuff" of life lived—and lay each gently on the floor. "The world comes to us through our senses," she said. "Choose an object that speaks to you and write about it. Start with what's there and just go. Allow yourselves to go to the dreaming place. Don't worry about the form; it will take care of itself. Writing is about telling the truth, not manipulating the material. Just let the words come. We'll write for twenty minutes."

I leaned forward and scanned the array of objects, certain that nothing on the floor had anything to say to me. I fingered a ring of keys, wondered if anyone would take the crucifix, then chose a half-empty pack of

Camel cigarettes and returned to my seat. I smelled the stale tobacco and let my fingers trace the camel pictured on the cover. Suddenly, my mind was flooded with long-forgotten images. I picked up my pen and began to write, memories of my father spilling out onto the page, his obsession with cigarettes, the first spark of the matches, riding in his old Chevrolet pickup together, his cigarette always lit, his easy chuckle, his death from lung cancer.

When our twenty minutes ended, I was breathless. Pat asked if anyone would like to read aloud. My heart was pounding as I tentatively raised my hand. "I'll go," I said softly. I began reading, hearing my words move from my the page and into the air, hearing my voice gain strength, feeling the lump in my throat intermingle with the sheer excitement of taking my writing into the open. I was making my declaration. I was a writer.

Dad. I think he tried them all: Lucky Strikes, Marlboros, and Camels. First he smoked the ones without filters. Later, he switched. In the last few years, he went to several types of "lites," but it didn't matter. He just smoked more frequently and drew harder on each breath to satisfy his craving for nicotine.

But there were fonder memories: Dad driving all of us to Southern California, pulling an all-nighter so we wouldn't have to find a motel. In those days, my parents didn't have enough money for overnight stays. I kept vigil during the dark quiet of the night, another pair of eyes on the road as I sat in the front seat with Dad while the rest of the family slept. We shared something silent, something special between us.

As we drove, Dad lit up one cigarette after another. How I loved the smell of that first match strike and the meeting of flame and tobacco: it was an exotic perfume that belonged only to my father. Now I cannot stand the smell of cigarettes.

I remember him: the bulge in his shirt pocket, the fliptop box, the yellow stain on his fingertips, the spark of the match, that first deep inhale. . . . Then he'd relax, smile, and more likely than not, begin telling an embellished story from his childhood. I didn't care if it was fact or fiction. It was Dad's. He made me laugh. I loved him.

When they discovered the lung cancer, it had invaded his body. Just three months to live, said the doctor. And yet he smoked on. As November neared, and autumn turned toward winter, he'd don a wool stocking cap, bundle himself up in a blanket, wheel his oxygen tank out to the patio (Mom had long forbidden cigarettes in the house in a futile attempt to get him to quit), and light up a cigarette. Many of my last conversations with Dad were on the patio in those cold November days. Leaves fell, the air chilled, and winter stood in the wings, ready to make an entrance. Dad smoked on and withered away, growing smaller and more fragile each day.

Thanksgiving Day, 1992. Dad begged me to make the trip north for the family celebration, but that year, I didn't come, heartsick from the painful sibling dynamics my father's inevitable death had produced. I begged off. I'd come the week after Thanksgiving, I told him.

On Thanksgiving Day, my sister said, he'd finally gotten the strength to get out of bed and join the family at the dinner table. He called his grandson to help him put on his slacks, now drooping on his frail slender body, and cinched them tight with the white patent leather belt my sister and I abhorred. He sat down for his Thanksgiving dinner and had two helpings of everything, even two pieces of pumpkin pie. That night, unlike all the ones before, he didn't have a cigarette. He was too weak to wheel his oxygen tank outside; his breathing had become too labored to allow him to inhale. Instead, he sat in the old brown recliner in the family room, his regular place, and drank a double Jack Daniels. "That was a mighty fine meal, Mom." He raised his glass in a compliment to the cook. That night, my father died in his sleep.

Damn it Dad, I never got to say goodbye.

I finished reading and sat in silence as I received the affirmations of the group, what they liked; what stayed with them. I cannot remember what was said to me. I only remember that I felt all the nerve endings in my body come to life. I was on fire. This simple act of retelling my life experience in writing catapulted me into a new realm of creative self-expression and self-discovery. It gave me a way to relive and reframe my life. It gave me permission to tell my stories. It also helped me come to terms with my own cancer experience.

Although it had been only three weeks since I'd completed radiation, I did not reveal anything about my breast cancer experience to the group. It was only on the last day, in a short, timed exercise, that it finally made its way to the surface, surprising me when it did.

Pat read aloud a selection of beginning lines, all quotations from other writers. I chose one about going to bed alone and quickly wrote a light-hearted poem. As I finished, I looked at my watch and saw I still had seven or eight minutes left to write, so I chose another of the quotations, "The hospital corridor was dimly lit" and began writing. My pen moved rapidly across the page. I placed the period at the end of the final sentence just as Pat told us our time was up. My cancer journey appeared out of nowhere.

> The hospital corridor was dimly lit—or was it? Maybe it was the cast of the yellow walls, making the room seem eerie and unreal. Maybe it was just that it was not real: any moment now I would awaken from this yellowed, faded dream.
>
> I turned left into the waiting room. A montage of faces greeted me: men, women, a young teenage girl, a grade-school boy. Some with hair; some without. At least I didn't have to go through chemotherapy.
>
> I'd joined a private club, meeting each day at 3 p.m. Membership requirements were pale blue hospital gowns, 15-20 minutes of daily radiation, and some form of the "C" word invading your body.
>
> "Ms. Bray?" The cheerful voice jolted me into awareness. My name was being called. I looked up. It was me. This was happening to me. I nodded acknowledgment and smiled woodenly. Holding

the sides of my blue gown together, I stood and followed her down the yellow corridor.

I returned home from the workshop in a state of elation and promised myself I would continue to write and study writing. I enrolled in numerous creative writing workshops. I filled dozens of notebooks with poems and prose. I bubbled over with enthusiasm whenever anyone asked me what I was doing in the months following my treatment. I was alive again.

A Letter to My Sister

By Marcia Davis-Cannon

Dear Connie,

I remember how hard you took the news of my breast cancer. You were the one with the lumpy breasts and calcifications. You were the one who never had babies of her own to breast-feed. You were older. It didn't seem right for a younger sister to get cancer when you were still under observation, almost as wrong as a parent having to bury a child.

Now the doctors have found a lump in your breast.

Oh Connie, every nerve ending in the breast I have left jangles with that news. I would gladly have had all the lumps for this generation of our family and all the generations to come. I want to reach out across the miles and enfold you in a lopsided, bosomy hug. I know the sick, hurting fist-in-the-gut feeling of this news.

And yet, I somehow want to share with you the impact breast cancer has had on my life. I want to introduce you to laugh-with-you, cry-with-you nurturing of fellow survivors. Perhaps the sky has always been this blue, but now I revel in its blueness. The sun is warmer now, spring blossoms more fragrant, friendships more dear. Life has never been so precious.

Love,
Marcia

5

A Personal Journey of Writing and Healing

I turned to what I had always found most healing. Writers don't choose their craft, they need to write in order to face the world, and this was still true for me.
ALICE HOFFMAN

My Notebook, My Friend

Writing has always been an integral part of my life, the way in which I explored my own feelings and beliefs. As an idealistic teenager, I wrote and contemplated the meaning of life. I carried small, spiral-bound notebooks with brightly colored covers wherever I went. I chose my ink carefully, preferring in those youthful days purple to the more commonplace black or blue. My little notebooks were full of observations and questions. As a child, I was deeply religious, and I looked for signs of God in every corner of life. In one of my little books that survived my growing up and many moves, I wrote, "Last night, I looked at the moon and saw this . . . ," followed by a rough sketch of a full moon, its beams of light radiating out from it like a giant cross. Was it, I wrote on the narrow, blue-lined pages of my yellow notebook, a sign? I now realize I had confused the reflection through the window screen as the moon's own. At the time, however, I felt something magnificent had been revealed to me, that I was on the tip of a deeper discovery. I think that what mattered most, in those early years, was that I was trying, in those purple-inked musings, to make sense of life and all its mystery through writing. My writing practice had taken root and would sustain me for many years to come.

My family lived in a small Northern California town, Yreka, where one's spirituality was daily inspired by the dominating view of Mount Shasta, one of the more beautiful extinct volcanoes in the Cascade range. I did not know it at the time, but Mount Shasta has long been considered a spiritual or sacred site, first by the Native Americans who inhabited the vast wilderness over which the mountain reigned, and later by religious sects and new-age spiritualists. Perhaps, growing up in this extraordinarily beautiful landscape, my spiritual life had the opportunity to be experienced, to deepen. Perhaps, in the act of writing down my questions and thoughts, I was plumbing the depths of my own young soul and charting a life course of self-reflection, healing, and spiritual practice through writing.

I was a habitual journal keeper through college and into my adult life. If I had no journal, I would write on scraps of paper or backs of lecture notes and later paste the pieces into my writing notebook, many of which have survived a number of cross-country moves. Writing was the vehicle by which I explored my emotions, my successes, and more often, my disappointments, trying to understand where I had erred or misstepped, how I might have constructed an experience differently, what I had learned from my mistakes. Years later, as I returned to school to complete my doctorate in applied psychology, I would discover Donald Schön's work on critical self-reflection and the growth of professional skill. Writing had always given me the mechanism for self-reflection, whether personal or professional. I would incorporate the use of self-reflection as part of my research methodology as I outlined, researched, and wrote my doctoral dissertation.

In the summer of 1978, my writing was once again fueled by life upheaval. My marriage was disintegrating, and I sought to explore the confusion and chaos through journaling. Each morning and evening, I wrote furiously, replaying events, trying desperately to make sense out of the morass of emotion I felt, challenging my faith in the horrible pain and loneliness I encountered. I took refuge in my writing. It became a catharsis.

Writing in my journal, while it provided temporary relief, did not completely heal the hurt—at least not in pages of emotional venting between the black covers of my notebooks. But it provided the space and solitude to pour out my feelings, helping me, perhaps, to not overload my friends and family with my daily outpourings of grief and pain.

My emotional life intensified. In the midst of our separation, my husband drowned in the lake at his parents' farm. Nothing I wrote on the many pages of my journal could help me answer the questions that pummeled my heart and mind each night. I wrote myself in circles after my husband's death, and it was only in the act of combining traditional nondirective therapy (the safety of uncensored and nonjudgmental emotional expression) with writing poetry and creating stories from dreams, stories of our life together, and finally, his death as story, that I was able to move on from the continual repetition in my journals. That work was extraordinarily healing, life affirming, and affirming of my own creativity.

In the two years of therapy, my journal writing began to change as I talked through my life's upheaval and my emotions each week to a sympathetic listener. I began to capture my life struggle and the therapeutic relationship in poetry. Each week, I would write a poem, take it to my therapy session, and read it aloud to my therapist. He treated my poems as if they were gifts and never tried to interpret or dig beneath the imagery for deeper meaning. He simply made it safe for me to write and to take my writing beyond the privacy of my notebooks. I now realize how very important that safety was for my writing to flourish. Tess Gallagher, writing in her essay "The Poem As a Reservoir for Grief," said, "Poems have long been a place where one could count on being allowed to feel in a bodily sense our connection to loss." I wrote more than one hundred poems during my two years of therapy, poems that told my story of loss, grief, and recovery.

I now read some of the poems I wrote during that period and realize that, as poetry, many might be too laden with my own personal emotion. Some have possibilities. Some are already good. But I wasn't writing to become a literary giant. I was writing to work my way into understanding: of love, life, death, and my relationship to each. Writing in the context of therapy as I did during those many months facilitated and strengthened my emotional healing.

The death of my first husband catapulted me into new growth and self-development. I went back to school and earned a doctorate. I launched a fast-track business career. I wrote, but irregularly. My executive life was taking up my time, and it was filling every corner of my life. I was losing touch with my soul and myself. A self-acknowledged workaholic, I was miserable and yet unable to break my own self-destructive cycle, so internalized was my need for achievement and proof for myself that I could be successful in that fast-paced, demanding world. I finally resigned from my corporate executive position with an international career services firm in New York City and spent several months quietly rediscovering my hopes, my dreams, and myself.

During this period, my journals took on a different look and feel. I now invested in blank books, roller ball pens, and colored pencils. I wrote pages each day, unpacking the frustration and unhappiness I'd felt for several years. At the end of each writing session, I would draw a cartoon with my ink pen, a caricature of myself or some aspect of the life I was leaving behind, and carefully color it in with my multicolored pencils. In doing so, I turned frustration and anger into humor, recasting my emotions through the simple little cartoons. I was healing, regaining my sense of humor and perspective. My illustrated journals of 1997 remain among my most favorite.

I turned to my journals again for solace in 1999 as I struggled with the challenges of downsizing the not-for-profit I now led. My notebooks became collections of questions, proposed strategies, feelings, illustrations, and deep self-questioning, all reflecting the personal struggles inherent in leading in tough times. It was, as I mentioned earlier, in the midst of this protracted organizational decline that I discovered I had a form of early-stage breast cancer.

Freeing the Writer Within: Diagnosis to Discovery

Keep the artist within you alive and well.
LYNN RHODES'S *inscription in a book to me*

The experience of cancer, no matter how small or great, leaves an indelible mark on an individual. My diagnosis of breast cancer was a complete surprise. I had no symptoms. The day I made my way to the medical clinic for my annual exam in late April 2000, I did not suspect how dramatically my life was about to change. During my mammogram, the technician requested that several additional photographs be taken. I gave permission and submitted to a dozen or so more episodes of having my breasts flattened and pinched between the glass plates. I was not alarmed. I had once been told by a physician that my breasts were "very active," and additional photos during an exam were routine for me. This day would be different.

The mammogram examination revealed some calcifications in my left breast. More photographs were taken. The radiologist met with me, pointed to the suspicious areas on the photographs, and explained what it might mean. I heard nothing. She quickly arranged for me to be sent across the office complex to a surgeon for a second opinion. A short time later, I left the surgeon's office with an appointment for a biopsy the following week. I felt a flutter of nervousness, but dismissed it. Several days after the biopsy, I returned to hear the results, sitting as the surgeon explained the findings. It wasn't too bad. A ductal carcinoma in situ, he said, and he felt confident that a combination of lumpectomies, radiation, and tamoxifen would cure me completely.

I didn't hear the word "cancer" that afternoon, and I have no idea whether or not he actually used the "C" word. It was all a dream as far as I was concerned, a distraction from the pressures that confronted me at work. I sat patiently as he described the treatment options. He spoke carefully, but his words weren't making any sense to me. I waited for him to finish. I had few questions. I smiled and rose. I was late for a meeting and anxious to leave. Dr. Gregg held the door open and looked at me quizzically. "Are you all right?" he asked.

"Oh yes, I'm fine," I answered.

"Sharon, I'd like you back here tomorrow at 4 p.m. with your husband." He was firm.

"All right," I agreed pleasantly. "We'll be here."

The seriousness of it all began to sink in the next afternoon. I watched my husband frown as he listened to the surgeon, heard his questions, heard the doctor repeat what he'd told me the day before, heard his description of high-grade cells: "a very bad act," he said, if left untreated. Still I was numb. I read an article on breast cancer that evening.

"John," I called to my husband. "He said carcinoma, didn't he?" My husband nodded. "That's cancer," I exclaimed, my eyes wide with fear and sudden understanding.

John nodded again, "Yes, that's cancer."

I went to bed and lay awake most of the night.

I would quickly come to feel that I was lucky. My cancer had been diagnosed early, and it was noninvasive. That was good. It slowly began to dawn on me that I had been given an important message about my life. For years, I had been caught in a cycle of stress, burnout, and unhappiness, and while I acknowledged the pressure-cooker symptoms, I seemed to be able to do little to stop the escalating spiral of stress I was living. My longtime friend Lynn Rhodes, who teaches at Pacific School of Religion, was one of my lifelines.

In 1997, I returned from a three-and-one-half-year stint as a corporate executive in New York City, burned out and miserable. It was Lynn who encouraged me to consider signing up for the summer session creative writing workshop with Pat Schneider. "I believe you have more creations in you than you know," she wrote. But I was perpetually busy, and I never quite found the time. Invariably, I would leave my application unsent or, as I did in 1999, forfeit my registration fee.

Cancer changed all that. A few weeks after my surgery, in mid-May, I was in the radiologist's office after a round of radiation therapy. He asked how I was doing. "Fine," I said, treating the radiation therapy as incidental and moving on to tell him what I was really worried about: the difficult task of downsizing the nonprofit organization where I was CEO. He

52 | A Healing Journey

listened, nodding his head sympathetically. Then he extended his hand and gently touched my knee as I sat dangling my legs from the edge of the examination table. "Sharon," he said softly, "you need to learn to make yourself the most important priority for a while." I felt the lump in my throat and fought back my tears. "Yes," I said, "I know I should. I just don't know how to do it."

I left his office, got in my car, and drove south on I-280, headed for my office. I was only five minutes away from the building when I was overcome with sorrow. "How," I wondered aloud, "did I get so far from myself?" I pulled off onto the shoulder near Foothill Expressway. Moments later, I picked up my cell phone and dialed the number of the chair of my board. "I'm resigning," I told her. By the end of the week, I had signed up for Pat Schneider's workshop at GTU and called my friend Lynn to tell her I would need a place to stay for a week in August. Little did I know that my life would be forever altered by the experiences of that spring and summer.

A Journey Through Breast Cancer
By Judy Finney

The first wake-up call, the discovery of a lump, diagnosis: ductal carcinoma.

The relief of early detection and lumpectomy. Eight cancer-free years, each year marked as a milestone. Then comes the slow awareness of developing changes within the existing scar tissue. Nothing seen on mammograms so it must be imaginary, right?

Eventually the changes become more visible and can no longer be ignored, wished, or prayed away. Cancer again pounds on the door with both fists, loud and hard.

Diagnosis: massive invasive lobular carcinoma.

The heart-wrenching reality of a mastectomy, but that is not enough. Another surgery to remove muscle down to the chest wall. Six months of aggressive chemotherapy, hair loss, chemo brain, weight gain, depression, the interminable waiting. Lessons learned, loves renewed, friends made, tears shed together.

Support found with fellow sufferers and within my own heart by sharing the journey. Reconstruction looms near, what to do? What to do? What about the remaining breast? How much time before it is invaded with cancer? This is not an option that I can live with. I will sacrifice my innocent breast to the insatiable cancer monster and receive a reconstructed body.

And continue along the learning path to discover how to best use this gift of continued life that has been given.

6

From Pilot to Program

I am not sure where I read about the workshop, but it leapt off the page and I called immediately to enroll. I thought it sounded exactly right as a therapy for working out the life-changing nature of my diagnosis.

JEAN

The first ten-week pilot began in the spring of 2001 under the title "Writing and Healing." Offered on alternate Wednesday evenings, the original session ran for two hours. I introduced myself on the first evening to a group of a dozen women, all of whom had one thing in common: breast cancer. What the exact nature of their experience was, or at what stage they were in treatment or recovery, was unique to each woman. Yet the experience, no matter how small or great, bound us all together. Breast cancer had altered our lives in profound ways. I felt an undeniable humility that I had gotten off so easily with my own diagnosis and treatment. As I came to know the women and their extraordinary struggles with breast cancer, it was hard to think of myself as a "survivor." Yet I was grateful that I had experienced cancer and some of its treatments, for it provided me with a credibility and common language with the women that I might otherwise not have had.

The journey through breast cancer from diagnosis to recovery, or sometimes death, is a long one. The women in our first writing group represented a variety of several different stages of the cancer experience. The women were each at different points in their cancer journey, but having cancer at any stage was a badge of membership in the group.

The motivations for attending the workshop were as diverse as the stages in their respective journeys. Some were curious. Some, like Ann, felt there was more for them to learn from their cancer experience. "I wanted to use my breast cancer experience to learn more about myself," she said. Others, like Marcia, came because she used writing to help herself deal with her cancer and her mother's loss to the disease. "I . . . signed up immediately because I love to write, journaled through my cancer and my mom's. . . . I felt the need to write again."

Other women were facing either the beginnings or aftermath of treatments: lumpectomies, mastectomies, radiation, chemotherapy—and simply felt that the experience of writing could help them work through this time of life challenge and change. Varda, who would later lose her battle to breast cancer, was matter-of-fact: "I . . . found a flyer at the radiology waiting room. I like to write and felt this might be a positive way to deal with my cancer experience."

In the first pilot group, only one of the women, Wendy, was diagnosed with metastatic cancer. As a physician, Wendy knew well the prognosis she faced. She had only a few months to live. The mother of two teens, she came to see if writing would help her face the death sentence she had been given.

And so we began. I was excited, and I was nervous despite the fact that I was an experienced teacher and counselor. I had facilitated many adult groups, counseled hundreds of individuals in transition, written, published, and become a "cancer survivor" myself, but I had never before led a writing group.

I played it safe. In the first few sessions, I followed the format and exercises described in Pat Schneider's earlier book, *The Writer As an Artist*, and replicated a good deal of my first workshop experience with her.

The women shared my nervousness in our first few sessions. I have come to appreciate, many writing groups later, timidity and apprehension as normal in the beginning. Writing and sharing your work out loud takes courage. As a leader, I invariably experience a little wave of stage fright just before beginning a new writing group, wondering, Will it work as beautifully this time? It always does. Apprehension quickly gives way to relief, and then excitement takes over. Ann, a therapist and breast cancer survivor, had experienced writing as "hard work." Fearful of not writing well, she entered the group determined to keep her writing to herself. Her timidity was short-lived. Ann began to feel connected to the other women, and as she did, she ventured into the open, reading aloud and receiving the affirmations, at first with disbelief, then with unabashed gratitude and smiles.

During the pilot, I was slow to confront cancer directly in the writing exercises I offered to the women. It may have been my own timidity in leading a writing workshop as well as an overabundance of sensitivity to the women in the room that caused me to shy away from confronting cancer—and all its implications—head-on. Whatever the reluctance, I did not focus explicitly on it in the pilot sessions. I chose to concentrate more on encouraging the members' creative self-expression in writing. Yet, no matter what verbal prompt or writing exercise I used, it was the women's experience with cancer that they expressed. Cancer is not shy, nor the experience of it, and the women wrote about what occupied their greatest fears and kept them awake at night. Cancer came unbidden, right into the open, each woman's struggle with it begging to be shared with the group. Even then, as the group leader, I kept the writing prompts neutral, circling around the elephant in the room: cancer, recurrence, and death.

Throughout our first few sessions, Wendy, who told us so frankly that she had only a few months to live, kept her writing to herself. She was faithful in her attendance, appearing each week, increasingly frail, with thinning hair that gradually all fell out, and skin slowly taking on the pallor of jaundice. She wrote diligently in response to every single writing prompt and exercise, but she declined every opportunity to read aloud. "I'm not creative like the rest of you," she would say. "I'm really a technical writer." No amount of encouragement would sway her. We accepted her silence but continued to offer her the opportunity to read aloud. Just as routinely, she quietly declined. Then, five sessions into the pilot, it all changed, and I saw, firsthand, the healing power of writing—and reading aloud to a supportive community of others.

I began the evening with a guided imagery and a verbal prompt I had modified from a poetry exercise. "Imagine someone close to you," I instructed the group. "As if you were behind a camera, move into a close-up and focus on their hands." I invited them to observe the details of the hands: color, skin, fingers, and what the hands were doing. "Now," I suggested, "pull back to the long shot and see the person again. You have come to them with a question. Ask your question, and, when you are ready, begin writing. We will write for twenty minutes."

At the end of the timed writing, I asked, "Who would like to read aloud?" Wendy responded immediately. "I'll read," she said. I heard a quiet but discernible collective inhale of breath. Everyone in the room was surprised. We all leaned forward and waited as she began reading aloud to us.

She had written a portrait of her teenage son's hands, bruised and bloodied from practicing on his bass so often. Her son, who, when she saw him on stage playing with his band at his high school, rolled his eyes back in his head to be "oh so cool" and who, she realized, had grown taller and needed a new suit. Her son who would go away to university on the East Coast in the fall. Her firstborn. Yet she never could find the right time to ask him her question. Her question? Would he be all right, she wondered, when she was gone?

Hands
  By Wendy Klee

Hands with long, strong fingers for their size, but not really large. Nails short, not always clean. What do you expect of a teenage boy? Mid- and index fingers on the right hand sometimes blistered from playing the bass for eight hours straight after not having played for ten days, from playing extra hard to make up for having forgotten the cords to his amplifier. Playing the upright bass in youth symphony with a bow. Looking so serious and concentrating so hard. More often playing jazz without the bow and hooked up to the amplifier. On stage with the Gunn Jazz Band in his suit which is finally too short and now too tight. We must get him a new one before the last concert, but when? So "into" the music and concentrating so hard that it looks from the audience as if his eyes have rolled back into his head. Or, playing the electric bass, looking oh so cool.

What I want to know is almost impossible to ask, especially now as all the pressures and activities of senior year culminate. Interrupting bass practice would be annoying, and he has so little time for it now. Interrupting while he's madly writing out Physics or Calculus—not the right time. Rough-housing with his younger sister—not the right time for this question. The question? Will you be all right when I'm gone? Are we making a huge mistake sending you three thousand miles away to college, when it's almost guaranteed I'll die just before you start or during your first semester? The answer? I don't know, can't know, until the time comes.

Wendy began to weep softly as she read the last few lines of her piece. My own eyes were red with tears, and I saw several of the women dabbing at their eyes with tissues. We were all overcome with emotion, many of us mothers ourselves, many of us all too aware of the fine line between life and death that metastatic cancer signifies, and all of us acutely aware of Wendy's terminal state, for she had communicated her condition unemotionally and factually at the beginning of the workshop.

As she finished, a hush fell over the group, then I leapt in to respond, "Oh Wendy, that was just beautiful," and somehow, we all found our tongues and began to tell her what we liked, what was strong, and what stayed with us in her writing. I watched as she received the affirmation and affection from the group, watched as her cheeks flushed red and a smile broke across her pale face. From that evening on, Wendy read aloud every chance she got. Her memories and stories tumbled out in piece after piece of writing: the dollhouse she had as a child; the Macintosh apples she picked with her father; the story of her marriage told through all the curtains that decorated her windows over the years. She wrote from that evening on about a life lived and a life about to end, about her children and her hopes for them, about her anger at her cancer and her sorrow in having to leave her loved ones so soon. And when we joined hands at the end of each evening, she held onto our hands tightly and received the warmth and affection of the group.

On the way home from the writing workshop several evenings later, I reflected on the change in Wendy and remembered something I'd read in the research on writing and healing, about the necessity of going to the places that hurt the most or are the most difficult to write about and finding the courage to open those up. Cancer was part of our lives, and in confronting our greatest fear of it, as Wendy had done, a rich wellspring of memory and imagery was released. Her writing became more vivid and powerful, but she, too, was transformed. After weeks of watching her sit stiffly in the circle, her face tight and reluctant to read, we saw her now lean forward, eager to read aloud and respond to others' writing. One evening, after someone's particularly humorous piece, she threw back her head and laughed joyously, something I had never seen her do before. Perhaps, I thought, this is what is meant by the healing power of writing. She could not stop her death by writing, but she could tell her stories, share her experience, write her fears, and find a semblance of acceptance and peace. We all observed a new energy in Wendy as she wrote about the people she loved and relived so much of her life in the stories she shared.

When the second series began several weeks later, Wendy was there, but she only attended the first two sessions. When a woman misses more than one session in a row, I call to find out if she is all right. I was concerned about Wendy's absence and telephoned her at her home. She answered immediately. "We've been worried about you," I said. "We've missed you. . . ."

"Oh, Sharon," she replied, "I'm badly jaundiced now, I don't think I'll be coming back."

The following Wednesday, we wrote for Wendy, using one of our writing exercises to write letters to her, each of us telling her how important she had been to us, admiring her courage and her gifts of story, and expressing our fondness for her. We placed the letters in a three-ring binder as a gift from the group. I mailed it the next day.

Barely two weeks later, Wendy's husband called to tell me she had died. There would be a memorial service the following Sunday, he said, and would I come? "The writing group meant so much to her," he said. "It would be nice if you could be there."

I shared the news of Wendy's death with the women the following Wednesday evening, and we took time to be silent together. Several women were crying. Some held each other's hands. The loss of a member who had struggled so courageously brought our fears out into the open, and with it, a diminishment of hope. Our hearts were heavy that night. I didn't realize it then, but Wendy was teaching me a lot about what it means to be the leader of a writing group for women who are struggling with cancer.

The following Sunday I made my way to Wendy's home, where the memorial service was to be held. A small group of family, friends, and professional colleagues gathered in her backyard. I met her son as I came into the garden and introduced myself. He had flown home from Harvard, where he was enrolled in his first semester of coursework. I noticed that he was clutching the small booklet of the women's writing we had published from the first ten-week series. Three of Wendy's submissions were in it, including the piece she had written about her son's hands. "I'm going to read one of my mother's stories," he told me, "but not the one about my hands; I wouldn't be able to get through that one." Neither, I thought, could I.

The service was simple. It was an early autumn afternoon and the garden was bathed in warmth, flowers, and sunlight. Family members, friends, and colleagues stood to tell their remembrances of Wendy, paying tribute to her many contributions, selfless service to her patients, and love of her family. Her son took his turn in the center of the gathering and told the guests a little about his mother's writing. Then he read one of her stories, a remembrance of a screen door in her childhood. Her father and mother smiled, remembering the screen door too, perhaps for the first time in years. I stood quietly and felt Wendy's presence everywhere that day, and I understood that the stories she had so fervently written in all the weeks of the writing group were also a legacy of her life that now could be kept, read, and treasured by the people she loved. At the end of the second series, we dedicated our collected writings to Wendy and reprinted the piece about her son's hands, honoring her life and her gifts to the group as one of its members.

Wendy was a teacher to me in the last weeks of her life. A writing group leader must always be able to learn from her group members and continually refine and improve her approaches. One of Wendy's enduring gifts was in helping me to make the workshop experience more specific to the unique needs of the women who were struggling with breast cancer.

At the conclusion of the first pilot, while Wendy was still writing with us, I asked the women to evaluate the workshop experience. Everyone was enthusiastic and grateful, but Wendy encouraged me to become more courageous with the writing prompts. "We need to go there, Sharon," she said, "right into the heart of the cancer experience. We need to explore the darkness of it."

I acted on her feedback and changed my writing workshop process during the second series. I kept many prompts from the original pilot, but I created new ones that invited the women to confront and express directly their experience of cancer. Each evening now included an exercise that opened up some aspect of the cancer experience—for example, the fears that cancer produces, or the experience of hair loss, loss of one's breasts, surgery, scars, diagnosis, life before and life after cancer. The prompts unleashed a dam of memories and associated emotions: anguish, grief, fear, loss, laughter, and tears.

One evening, for example, I read Raymond Carver's poem, "Fear," aloud to the women and invited them to write about their own fears associated with cancer. Margaret's was a particularly powerful portrayal of the raw emotion associated with her diagnosis and struggle with a very aggressive form of breast cancer. When she read it aloud, the women were silent for a few moments before responding. Margaret's poem struck a responsive chord in everyone, expressing what many of them also felt and had not been able to say.

Fear

By Margaret Prien

Fear of recurrence
Fear of dying
Fear of radiation complications
Fear of more radiation burns
Fear of skin grafts
Fear of infection
Fear of osteoporosis
Fear of another fracture
Fear of dependence
Fear of not being here
Fear of not seeing Marcelo
Fear of never regaining my balance
Fear of visual impairment
Fear of the numbness in my hands & feet never going away.
Fear of skin burning in the sunlight
Fear of a loss of energy
Fear of crying during media interviews
Fear of not accomplishing goals
Fear of not remembering
Fear of chemo-brain
Fear of not finding a cure soon enough
Fear of missing the joy of living
Fear of pain
Fear of not seeing grandchildren
Fear of missing Kathleen's wedding
Fear of the next mammogram
Fear of the next nuclear bone scan
Fear of never being the same person
Fear of no bad hair days
Fear of time passing swiftly
Fear of not being brave at the end
Fear of missing life.
Fear of the nightmare never ending

Writing about the impact of cancer enhanced the women's ability to write about all aspects of their lives. Going into the darkness and facing it down, naming it and bringing it into the open freed the women to write more vividly and powerfully about other life experiences, as witnessed in Wendy's writing after she so poignantly expressed her fear of confronting her death with her son. Now, during every writing session we experienced the full range of emotions as we read aloud what we had written. Our lives began to intertwine every evening in a deep and abiding intimacy of knowing: not only about one another's disease or struggle to survive it, but about parents, first dates, family rituals, taboos, marriages, grandparents, places—the full rainbow of life, of living.

One evening Carol Braunshausen wrote a descriptive piece about returning to her grandparents' farm in Illinois, where, as a child, she learned to ride a bicycle and sled on a small inclined street in front of their house.

> Ah, Illinois. Flat and flatter than flat . . . it was summer. The corn was tall and green. It went for miles, broken only by the occasional farm road or house. I stopped the car to use my new panoramic view camera. No one would believe how corn could go for miles. But to me, it was the way it should be. I was home.

"I love this group," Carol said excitedly as she finished reading aloud. "We're not only writing about cancer; we're writing about life."

Writing from our memories, as Patricia Hampl says, is a chance to live life twice. Carol's remembrance of a place she had loved as a child reminded us that, in the context of confronting a life-threatening illness, telling the stories of our lives through writing becomes all the more poignant and powerful.

Irena Olender's writing also shifted, moving to an earlier time in her childhood, a time during the Second World War, a time when she and her family endured the harsh environment of a concentration camp. Yet there was beauty, community, and gifts, and one evening, she remembered how it was to be four and receive a wonderful surprise in a time of suffering and poverty.

> Today is a special day, my mother has said. Today you are four! I know that birthdays are special. Most mothers in the camp are trying to make a celebration of some kind for the birthday children. So here I am, a little girl standing in a circle of smiling women and staring children, feeling self-conscious and awkward. . . .
>
> Today they hand me the present: an old flat tin can that used to hold cookies or crackers long ago, in a time unknown to me. The tin can is carefully covered with little pieces of cloth. I recognize small pieces and patterns of the old dresses women are wearing. . . .
>
> Inside the cloth-covered can are scraps of old cloth and fabric. On top of this little mattress, in this exquisite little cradle, lies my first little rag doll. Handmade, of course, out of whatever can be found in this barren environment . . . What does one do with such a treasure?

As the weeks progressed, the women's writing expanded into other areas of life and remembrance beyond cancer, and an unmistakable community began to form. The women expressed and experienced all the bonds of strong social glue: belonging, emotional safety, a common language out of the experience of cancer, and strong affection for one another. Writing together was truly therapeutic and deeply healing. Writing and sharing our stories aloud, receiving acknowledgment and affirmation from one another, having the shared safety to open up our emotions, and sharing the experience of cancer forged strong, supportive bonds between the women. They offered help to one another, advice, suggestions, and referrals to medical doctors. If a member was absent for any unexplained reason, they worried and reached out—the fear of recurrence or death always a possibility. We had become a powerful support group with writing at the center of the experience. At the conclusion of the pilot program, Carol Lyn Conragan described how she experienced the power and support of the writing group during her cancer treatment in a fantasy she titled "Warrior Women." The writer imagined herself in a jungle and coming upon a clearing:

> Women were dancing and singing around the fire, a contrast of sweet songs and spears thrust up into the sky. The women appeared fierce, but there was a quality of gentleness about them. . . . My heart nearly burst with sudden gladness when I recognized the women: my writing group members! I knew I was safe and would have help finding my way out of the dark jungle.

Change

By Candice Michel

I'm no stranger to change. She tracks me, dogging my every step, no matter how still I am or how quietly I tiptoe. Until finally, drowning in the stagnant stillness, I reach out to her and she suddenly vanishes, leaving me to frantically search for her disappearing shadow. I don't like her much. She's often strident, unyielding, and calls at the most inopportune moments, relentless in her need to disrupt my hard-won peace. And I'm sure she doesn't much care for me, angry, stubborn, with a sailor's vocabulary—all directed at her. But we're joined in this strange dance of life, unable or unwilling to pull free until the music finally slows, then stops. I need her for life and she depends on me to live. I have begun to notice that the rough edges, the angles and straight lines I took such pride in nurturing, are being rubbed soft and rounded, like a piece of sea-tumbled driftwood washed up on the sand. I hate her. I love her. She is my deadliest nightmare, and my sole salvation. It's hard to need her so much.

7

Writing Together

THE SCRIBBLING WOMEN OF CBHP

> I have been able to explore and share my hidden
> terrors, my hopes and joys with this compassionate
> group of women. With them I have laughed and
> cried, vented frustrations, confronted my fears and
> embarked upon the journey of healing.
>
> JUDY, writing group member

Learning from the Pilot

As we began our second series, a number of the women
were undergoing chemotherapy. The impact on the group
dynamic was unmistakable, for the aftermath of treatments
took a heavy toll on each individual. I remembered Wendy's
advice, and each evening I incorporated writing exercises that
directly addressed the cancer. Everyone's writing intensified,
revealing the raw emotion that underlies this disease. Ann Gifford's short piece, "Breast Cancer in Paris," reveals the underlying terror of a cancer diagnosis.

Breast Cancer in Paris
By Ann Gifford

All alone and scared
Wanting to whine
Be comforted

Held to someone's
Warm, copious
Bosom.
Will I die?
Out of control
Hopeless—nowhere
To hide from this terrible trap?
I can't cope with it.

Judy was one of the women undergoing chemotherapy when the second series began. She came to the writing group not only because she wanted to write, but because she wanted to use her writing to work through some of the pain and anguish of the cancer ordeal. She wrote about her experience of writing during her treatment:

When we are in chemotherapy, we are so very different from others. Here we can identify with each other. Everyone shares the experience. As you see others getting stronger, you realize that you are getting stronger too. Hearing other people's writing, how others have made it through this, gave me courage. The shared journey and knowing they have made it gives me hope. You know you will make it too. Getting stronger is not easy.

Ceci used her creative self-expression in art therapy after her first cancer diagnosis. When cancer struck a second time, she decided to try the writing group. "I wanted to use [writing] as a creative process for my healing," she said, even though she found writing to be a "very slow and painful process." She wrote, "It was a bold decision on my part to allow myself to share my experiences with others. . . . It's very helpful to talk and write about our fears, hopes, and dreams, knowing that we aren't alone, but are part of this universal experience."

Confronting the cancer experience head-on seemed to strengthen each woman's resolve to triumph over the disease. Scarves and wigs were shed within the first two or three sessions, revealing the smooth, round beauty of each woman's bald head. Judy Finney wrote about her hair loss one evening in response to Lucille Clifton's poem, "Hair."

Hair
By Judy Finney

As a child, I had curly red hair with a mind of its own.
As a teenager, all attempts to tame it failed miserably.
As I grew older, it gave up much of its curl and its bright red color, as if it had fought the good fight and was now resigned to "style."

After my first chemotherapy treatment my hair slowly disappeared. I gathered it up as it fell out, somehow trying to save it.
Finally, I threw it away and actually enjoyed the ease of "hairlessness."

Now, it has begun to grow in again, very slowly. It seems darker than I remember and I cannot tell if it will be curly again or not.
It is like slowly unwrapping a present,
and I am filled with anticipation over my new gift.

We not only wrote about hair—having it and losing it—we wrote about breasts: having them, losing them, and reconstructing them. We dove into our cancer journeys and spoke back. We voiced our fears, and we voiced our tenacity. We joined forces and voices—all in the act of writing. Neli Stascausky addressed her cancer directly one evening:

Cancer, you are malignant, unpredictably mean
but there is an army of us:
patients, doctors, friends,
working night and day to block
your way,

And I fervently believe
Someday we'll prevail.

During this second series, we dubbed ourselves "The Scribbling Women of CBHP," demonstrating the same gutsiness as the literary women Nathaniel Hawthorne so deplored. We were tough, tender, and tenacious women, and the healing power of writing together was unmistakable. The spirit of the writing group was described in an article in *The CBHP Report* in December 2001:

> Nathaniel Hawthorne once complained he could not get his own work noticed due to the power and dominance of the women writers of his day, a group he contemptuously referred to as the "damned mob of scribbling women." Nathaniel, be advised: every other Wednesday evening at CBHP, a similarly powerful group of women gather, not, perhaps to become literary giants, but as women possessed with a desire to write, to tell their stories, and to nurture their own creativity. These are the Scribbling Women of CBHP, a strong, courageous, and supportive community of writers who meet every other Wednesday for the creative writing workshop, "Stories of the Journey."

"The group experience sustained me through the worst year of my life," wrote Karen, who had come to the writing group in the midst of undergoing her chemotherapy regimen. "I felt heard, seen, validated, understood." Karen's short piece, "I Write Because," speaks to the power of her writing experience during her cancer treatment.

I Write Because
By Karen Usatine

I write because it makes sense of my experience.
I write because I love words, language, images, expression.

I write because it is not enough just to live life.

I write to relive the joy and sorrow, sometimes making
sense of the senseless.
Sometimes I write just to say, "I was here, and THAT
happened to ME,
and this is who I was, who I am, who I am becoming."
Witness, yes. To my own truth.
And to the experience of others.

I write because the multicolored passion,
the fire and ice, rage and joy cannot be silenced
within the life of one woman.
One frightened girl-child,
one shining warrior.

Ann, who had undergone a mastectomy only a year before, wrote:

I think I was wounded in a number of ways by cancer—losing .
. . my positive feelings about my body and my health. I lost a sense
of control over my life . . . feeling vulnerable increased my fears of
others and my trust. . . . I also felt alone. Writing together with
other women who had the same experience allowed me to express
my feelings about having cancer and have them validated. This was
healing. Being accepted as part of a group was healing for me too. .
. . I felt less alone.

Judy also reflected on her experience:

I was still in chemotherapy when I began, and I had been hit very
hard. It took me a long time to come to grips with it. Writing helped
me get the emotions out. . . . It helps me put it in perspective and
begin to deal with it better. Writing crystallized my thoughts and
feelings that I had trouble talking about. . . . When you read aloud

you hear things that you didn't even know were there. You've gotten to the truth, like a discovery . . . a revelation.

One evening I offered the women Elena Georgiou's poem "Questions in the Mind of the Poet as She Washes the Floors" as a writing prompt. Judy chose one question from the poem, "Can I be happy with the person I've become?" and wrote, describing her journey of pain, growth, and revelation.

Can I Be Happy With the Person I've Become?
By Judy Finney

I loved my life.
I was happy. I was focused.
I had given up a boring career and embarked upon one that I
    prized.
I had conquered fears, struggled, grown, learned from my mistakes.
I found a lump ten years ago, underwent a lumpectomy
and radiation, and survived, passed the test with flying colors!

I thought I was "home free," safe, and gone on with life.
I was optimistic about the future and my place in it.

Then cancer struck again.
Now, I have survived the ravages of mastectomies,
chemotherapy and reconstructive surgery.
My body healed, only the daily glimpses of scars
and numbness remind me of the physical toll taken.
But there was a dramatic shift in my psyche.
I was no longer the shining Pollyanna I once was.
I was now a different person whom I struggled to understand.
I lost confidence in my abilities and myself.
As I buried dear friends lost to this horrible disease,
I felt betrayed, no longer sure of the future.

Life was no longer a safe haven.

Slowly, tentatively, painfully, with time and the help of friends and
    lovers,
I've come to understand this new self.
I'm feeling healthy again and each new day is a gift for which I am
    grateful.
I treasure the simple pleasures that life has to offer and
am happy with the person I've become.

Clarissa agreed and added, "Writing with the other women who are
undergoing the same journey is a liberating one. The feelings just flow
out, and you don't edit your emotions. It gave me an excuse to be
human.... There are lots of others like me."

Clarissa speaks to an important aspect of the healing benefits of writing together. Not only were the women encouraged to confront and
write about their cancer journey, the safety and support of the group
environment allowed them to express their emotions associated with
their illness openly, without fear of recrimination or criticism, which is
one of the most important aspects of writing that is truly healing.

It was an important step in the journey of healing to write about
one's experience with cancer, but even more powerful was the act of
reading aloud, sharing each other's stories, of bearing witness, receiving,
and responding with affirmation and acceptance of one another. When
Ceci reflected on this part of her experience in the group, she said,
"Reading my writing out loud is an affirmation of my own experience.
Sharing my writing is an emotional release, a venting of my inner angst.
... I feel that I am in a safe environment with others who have also been
devastated emotionally or physically."

A Circle of Friends

As we came together week after week, one thing was unmistakable:
The act of writing together was life-affirming, joyous, and deeply inti-

mate. By the end of the ten meetings together, we had built a strong and vibrant sense of community. This had taken time to develop, but as the writing program matured, the social barriers seemed to vanish more quickly, and by the third session of our ten together, a community had begun to form. I observed a natural progression of "stages" in each series. In the first two to three sessions of each series, or the "introductory stage," we were becoming acquainted with each other and learning to trust the writing process. Several women would decline to read those first two or three meetings, while others would venture timidly into the open. By the end of the third meeting, the dynamic of the group had shifted, and the bonding of the group members was apparent. Deep emotions began to rise to the surface in the writing, and everyone became less self-conscious and more engaged in listening and responding to one another.

The safety of the group environment enabled us to go deeper, and in the responses to the exercises, we confronted more openly fears and feelings about cancer. At this stage, the women were more willing to dive beneath the water line to write and bring the pain and sorrow to the surface. When asked to write about what the experience of cancer had meant to each woman, Karen Jandorf's poem, "Someday I'll Be Grateful," revealed the vulnerability and complex emotions of a woman who lost both her breasts to cancer.

Someday I'll Be Grateful
By Karen Jandorf

If you touch my chest, you will feel my heart in your hand.
It is that close to the surface.
All its protective covering has been taken away.

If you hug me, you will feel my heart beat against your chest.
You will know the syncopation of my fear, my excitement, my equanimity.
There is no camouflage left.

If you see me, you will notice my shoulders fighting,
curling inward, stretching outward.
Conflicting desires to contract and expand.

If you sense me, you will feel my heart protecting itself.
It is too naked, too raw, too vulnerable.
Energetic armor created in the wake of exposure.

If you love me, though, you will invite me to unfold.
Your hand will become a safe haven for my broken-winged heart.
You will slowly and gently help me remove the suit of arms.
Your heart will become my polyrhythm and you will dance with
me.

Strong emotions often overtake many of the women as they read what they have written. We who listen are also moved to tears from time to time. Opening up to express the strong emotions associated with cancer is an important passage in writing about our experience and in healing. Equally important is the leader's ability to help the group be present and receive each woman's writing quietly, holding it as a fragile gift, not rushing to intervene, interpret, or comment, "Yes, I know just how you feel." In this way, we ensure that safety for the writer is kept intact.

A large box of tissues is placed on the center table every evening. In those moments of deep emotion, of shared experiences, in the affirmation and support of the group, we begin to find strength in ourselves. Healing occurs not only in the writing and reading aloud, but also in reaching out to help one another heal.

The women's strength and will to survive the ordeal of cancer was expressed in many different ways in their writing. They began to talk back to their illness and reframe how they thought of it in response to the different exercises. One evening, I asked the women to personalize their cancer, give it a voice, and then talk back to it directly. Marcia Davis-Cannon's determination to win her battle with the disease was evident when she wrote:

Hey cancer!
Leave my kids alone.
You got my mom.
You got my dad.
You tried your best with me.
Now leave my kids alone;
Just leave my kids alone!

I found it deeply gratifying as the leader to hear the strength emerging in the women's voices as they read aloud, see the shift in posture and body language as they felt the support of the group, hear them express surprise at what they had written, see the smile of satisfaction and delight as they received feedback, watch them respond to one another with warmth and acceptance.

We had begun to write about everything: memories, cancer, fantasies, dreams. Very soon, we were writing not only for our lives, but about our lives. Writing about our lives, as intimately and openly as we wanted, did something else for the group. It brought joy, laughter, poignancy, and a full range of rich story and memory to each writing session. The women shared an intimacy unlike any I had experienced before—all through writing. Perhaps Neli Stascausky expressed it best for all of us when she described her experience in the writing group:

When we gather together to write, the exterior world disappears, and we all reach inside our inner selves. Depending on the weight we experience in the different facets of our lives, we manifest ourselves in wonderful voices: an outpouring of vibrant, multicolor art comes out, sadness and happiness, darkness and light, pain and relief, warmth and cold, rainbows and clouds, laughter and tears. And at the end of each evening we part, and driving home I glide: happy, fearless, ethereal and eternal? Perhaps . . .

During the second series, the group became, as it now does during every ten sessions, a strong and important source of support and healing for the group members. Karen's enthusiasm for the writing group was unmistakable when she wrote, "It is the strength I get from knowing this group exists. The writing group is a safety net for me. There is nothing else like it in my life. It is so valuable. It is brimming over with exactly what I need. I get at least as much back as I give."

Irena echoed her appreciation for the support and community she experienced. "I haven't had good experiences with support groups; I didn't like them, but in the writing group I have found it wonderfully supportive and supportive of what I am trying to do. I liked that it didn't just deal with cancer; there is a whole other reality outside of cancer."

Writing and transforming experiences into stories and poems became a regular part of the women's lives, the importance of it undeniable in Jean's comment: "I have scheduled my life around this group. . . . In the short time I've been with the group, I have developed a network that doesn't end at the evening. I feel them when I go for the treatments."

"There is a wonderful strength in fighting a common enemy. . . . It is like warm and affirming friends who truly understand," Judy said. Yes, that was it. The group was more than a writing group. In the act of confronting their fears and struggles with cancer, they had become a strong and supportive community of women who gave each other strength to keep going, to survive and to heal.

During the second series, while I browsed shops on a Saturday afternoon, I found a candleholder called "Circle of Friends." I bought it immediately and carried it to the next writing group session. That evening, I quietly placed the candleholder in the center of the small coffee table in the meeting room. I put a large white candle in it as the women began to settle in their places to write. "When I saw this candleholder," I told them, "I was reminded so much of this group—your courage, your spirit, and your caring and support of each other." I lit the candle, watching the smiles on the women's faces, their heads nodding in approval. The whisper of an ancient campfire brushed against our memories. We had become a circle of friends, gathered together in the light of the candle, pens in hands, waiting to write together and share our stories.

Baring the Soul

By Karen Usatine

Breasts. Scars. Nipples. No nipples.
Smiles. Stares. Daring you to react.
Young. Old. Alone. Together.
Sisters. Lovers. Partners. Crones.

How universal yet unique the experience is.
What strength it takes to go on with life.
When will a semblance of security return?
Where does the grief go?
Why is there no early detection for all?

How can an epidemic remain so hidden?
What will the young girls find in their softness?
When can breasts be valued but not objectified?
Where is it written that symmetry is sacred?
Why is treatment more like torture?
Who will finally put a stop to all this madness?

8

When One Loss Begets the Memory of Another

What I was looking for during ten months of
chemotherapy and radiation was a way to make
sense out of sorrow and loss.
ALICE HOFFMAN

The women in my writing group were bound together by a
significant and traumatic life event: the diagnosis of breast
cancer. The emotions surrounding a cancer diagnosis and
treatment are complex and, at times, intense. Coming face to
face with one's own mortality, with the knowledge that something alien and destructive is inhabiting the body, that curing
it may mean fighting poison with poison, or the disfigurement of one's body—these are horrifying and deep challenges
of what a breast cancer diagnosis presents to an individual.
Alice Hoffman, herself a breast cancer survivor, wrote of her
illness in *The New York Times*. "Novelists know that some
chapters inform all others. These are the chapters of your life
that wallop you and teach you and bring you to tears, that
invite you to step to the other side of the curtain, the one that
divides those of us who must face our destiny sooner rather
than later."

Yet, whether our destiny would come sooner or later,
buried wounds began to surface among the women in the

group. Marcia found the first few sessions stirred up her feelings of loss.

> I had a lot going on when I started the class—my health issues, my mom's death . . . and a lot of those feelings had been bottled inside so I could be strong for my family. When I started the class, almost every writing exercise was a tearful one for me. . . . I felt the freedom to go deeper in my feelings and pour them onto the page because the environment was so affirming, encouraging, and accepting.

I have also had experience leading bereavement support groups, and I knew it was not uncommon that a new loss rekindled the memories and emotions of other losses. Indeed, when my own father died, my youngest daughter, Claire, could not bear to attend his funeral. Her father had died ten years earlier, when she was nine years old. Losing her beloved grandfather intensified her heartache. "I can't go, Mom. I can't," she told me when we packed the car to drive the 350 miles north to my parents' home. "I just feel like an orphan all over again."

Often the experience of cancer has the same effect. One loss begets the memory of another. The emotions of life struggles and losses from earlier times may be closer to the surface at a time we feel vulnerable and out of control of our lives. We tell our stories in order to survive, and in doing so, we remember, recover, and find some measure of control and healing over our past. An invitation to think about scars, seen or unseen, old or new, frequently evokes powerful writing. Scars tell stories; scars carry the memory of other losses or painful life events. We all have scars. Jean Allington wrote about hers:

Scars
By Jean Allington

> None of us are unscarred.
> There is childhood,

night fears.

Parents doing their scary but true best.

First love,

teenage angst.

Marriage, children, divorce,

separation, death.

Loss and scars,

scars and loss,

life and lessons.

Then there is cancer.

When we think we have seen it all,

learned the lessons, wizened by our mistakes,

thrilled by our triumphs.

We've survived life, we think.

Then there's cancer.

Life in a microcosm.

All the lessons,

all our wisdom,

all our youthful scars,

all the losses,

bundled up in tumor cells,

and lymph nodes.

Memory meets reality.

We start all over again

to live beyond the scars.

The love and support of others can help us heal from our wounds, help us accept and understand the scars of our bodies and spirits. The presence of a supportive community with shared experience contributes to our mutual support, our strengthening, our sense of belonging and well-being. "Facing down . . . certain death, only to confront it again in a similar form but a different place," said Susan Sontag in an interview in *The Guardian,* "forces a permanent re-evaluation of your sense of self. There is something about facing a mortal illness that means you never completely come back. . . . There's something in you that's permanently strengthened or deepened. It's called having a life."

Having a life also acknowledges that we continually face loss or the threat of it. Jean, who was struggling with metastatic colorectal cancer, wrote about facing down the threat of mortality, combining the experiences of a Midwestern farm childhood with the struggle of her life, in "Face-Off with a Pig."

Face-Off with a Pig
By Jean Allington

My good friend Jim always said, "Never wrestle with a pig: the pig likes it and you only get muddy."

I am facing off with a pig of a clinical trial, trying to make it a pet pig. I want to fatten it up, make it into a good-eatin' porker: tasty and succulent, not too lean, nourishing. There is no time to waste. I am, after all, already sick.

In the ring is the medical establishment of rules, closed records, little lies, wasted waiting time, asking the wrong questions of the wrong people, people providing services as though they are dishing slop into a trough.

I am already sinking into the mud, having spent eleven hours last week and eight hours so far this week on the phone, talking, wheedling, cajoling for appointment times, reports to be sent, films to be read, and bills to be paid. In addition, there is the time spent taking notes of the date and name of my contact at the insurance company, HMO, or the Medical Center. Information is doled out a piece at a time, not enough to fatten up this hawg. That doesn't count the twenty or so hours spent at doctors' appointments, taking tests, and having blood drawn. Then there is the time required for therapy and support groups to help me get through all this slop.

Wrestling with a slick pig is a tiring experience—we're talking about a full-grown hog here—hard for this already tired body. "No," I say, "I am not coming to the Medical Center for tests on my 'week off '." I must have caught the beast off-balance that time: It only took one protest, one phone call, and I won that round. I lost the round that would have allowed me to start the trial last month, when I was less ill. The battle for my precious time was already lost to the clinicians that raised this pig: It is eight weeks on treatment with only one week off in between for sixty-two weeks if all goes well. If not, I am out of the ring, maybe down for the count.

Writing together allows us to heal by giving us the opportunity to remember, reconstruct, and reflect on our pasts. In the timed writing exercises, I discovered that we were repeatedly surprised by where our writing might take us or by the emotions that welled up as we read aloud.

One evening, as I led the women in one of our favorite writing exercises, the prompt took one writer back to a disturbing remembrance from childhood. I asked them to imagine the photograph of someone close, explore the details in the photograph, and when they were ready, begin to write from the memory the photo evoked.

One woman described a father in what was, at first, a child's loving remembrance of a parent; a shadow, however, lurked in the background, and as she continued to write, the darker side to the father emerged in her writing. When she read aloud, we were gripped by a passage where, one terrifying night, the drunken father dangled a child's small body from a ship's deck out over open water. She faltered and paused to wipe the tears from her eyes. "I'd forgotten about that," she said. "I didn't know I was going there when I started writing." We all were silent for a moment, then I thanked her for her courage in writing and in reading, and we began to give her feedback: the passages we remembered, found strong, that we liked, affirming her writing and ensuring the safety for the revelation of life stories and emotional truths to be revealed.

Even as the leader, I sometimes feel a rush of emotion begin as old losses surface. In response to the same exercise of imagining a photograph of someone close to us, I wrote:

I stare at the photograph in my hand. September 1970. You are smiling, radiant with all the pride and excitement of a newly minted parent. You are a father. Your eyes are aglow with the unabated joy of holding your firstborn. She is nestled in your protective arms, asleep and oblivious to the pop of the flashbulb, and to the ear-to-ear grin of the young, dark-haired, bearded man who holds her forward to the camera.

We were so full of hope and promise then. I married my rebellion in you. Young, idealistic children of the sixties, we made our way to Canada the summer of 1968, driving across the vast continent in a tri-colored Rambler station wagon, something you bought from a Mexican farm laborer. "A fantastic deal," you said. All of our worldly goods were pulled behind in a U-Haul trailer. Bismarck, our Irish setter, sprawled out long in the back seat. Remember? We had to drive at night through the desert; the old Rambler engine overheated in the midday sun. It was our grand adventure.

Elinor will fly into San Francisco tomorrow. Your first daughter is a young accomplished woman of 30, full of promise and vitality. Sometimes, as she moves across the room, I see you in the way she holds her body, how she walks through a doorway, the way her shoes wear down on the inner soles, or even in the brand of political activism that is now her own. You're there, a presence, a ghostly shadow, a memory that floats up from these old photographs, a man, and my husband, who died beneath the murky waters of a small Indiana lake. I hear the echo of our young daughters' voices over the telephone that July afternoon in 1981. "Mommy, Mommy, come quick. The divers will get him, Mommy. The divers will get him. Come quick."

In the book *Writing and Healing*, Marian MacCurdy wrote, "We cannot recall a difficult memory without also re-experiencing the emotional charge it produces." The experience of this writing group—the acceptance, the lack of judgment or interpretation, and the safety in which to write—reminded me again that writing can be deeply therapeutic, yes, but a writing group does not exist for the purpose of therapy. A writing group exists to write—freely, openly, courageously, deeply, joyously—and the strong sense of community that evolves between us in the writing and telling of our stories allows us to articulate the meaning of our cancer experience and of our lives. It not only helps us get through our illnesses, other trauma or suffering, but to go beyond them: to heal.

Have I Loved Well in the Autumn of My Life?

By Neli Stascausky

Have I loved well the crisp invigorating mornings I walked
surrounded by trees
whose browning golden leaves falling to the ground
were carpeting my path?

Have I loved well the sunny blue-sky afternoons
that enlightened my mind
making me fly to the past rainbows of my life?

Have I loved well the warm and cozy nights
I spent in the comfortable arms of family and friends
that brought symphonic music to my heart?

Have I loved well my self, to let go of my doubts?
I want to say, Yes! I have.

9

Writing as Sanctuary

Through the exchange of stories, we help to heal
each other's spirits. . . . Isn't this what a spiritual life
is about?

PATRICE VECCHIONE

In a powerful piece begun in our writing group, "Journey into
a Dark Place," Carolyn Schuk wrote about

> a journey that I did not plan to take, and which I have
> not finished, and perhaps will never finish. . . . It is a
> journey into that geography where reality gives vocal
> and disquieting evidence that you may not keep the
> promises you made to yourself when you were twenty.
> . . . It is a place where you must relinquish your fate into
> the hands of a merciful God or perhaps to the whim of
> an uncaring universe. It is a journey on a downward
> path that leads to the foot of one's own personal cross,
> the one you must take up and carry into your own heart
> of personal darkness . . . . When you have been diagnosed
> with cancer, cancer writing becomes your prayer book,
> your daily office, and like a monk, you faithfully mark
> the liturgical hours of your involuntary vocation with
> the canticles and sacred texts of the cancer library.

Writing and Spirituality

Carolyn was referring specifically to her cancer writing as her prayer book, but she also touched upon the spiritual act inherent in writing. Pat Schneider, in *Writing Alone and With Others*, describes her own writing as "my primary spiritual discipline. Here, writing, I struggle to understand myself and my world. . . ." Writing, for Pat Schneider, "is my vocation, and my work is my prayer."

Writing, whether about cancer or other life experiences, is truly a meditative act. It can also be a deeply spiritual experience. Writing was important in some religious traditions. Journal keeping was a crucial means of recording life events and their religious significance. Our spiritual and emotional selves are inextricably linked. Writing allows for a deepening: looking to ourselves to gain insight. In listening to our hearts and spirits when we write, we have an opportunity to discover ourselves and our needs, and to embark on our own journey of personal and spiritual growth.

Our spiritual journey is intimately bound to our psychological and emotional journeys. A crisis such as breast cancer brings a reassessment of life and of our beliefs at the most fundamental level. In response to a writing prompt on fear, Varda Nowack Goldstein reflected on her experience of cancer, and in doing so, addressed her spirituality:

> I never cried for my mother when she died. There was no time, and there was no money. There was a continent between us. During the time she was ill, I could never visit. There was no one to take care of my children; no money for a plane ticket. She was gone, and I did not allow myself the time to mourn.
>
> I never cried for my father when he died. He had been gone for so long mentally. It was a hideous disease that took my handsome, jovial father and turned him into an angry old man. He died quietly in his sleep. "Woke up dead," they said, "a true blessing."
>
> I never cried for my sister when she died. The house was always

full of people, night and day. She always told us she would live. Even when we wrapped her left breast, a bleeding tumor, in gauze. She promised us she would live. And since she never spoke of death, we honored her wishes. In the end, she was angry with me. I served her tea that was too hot. Standing by her bed, just months after my father's death, I remembered her ripping the collar of her plain black dress at the gravesite, so clever and devout.

I never cried for myself when I lost my left breast. If I truly had faith, could I question my fate? I never prayed for my life. Did I have the right to ask for Divine Intervention?

I have been the model. I have done so well. I have never shown signs of depression. I have never asked, "Why me?" Perhaps I would be afraid of the answer.

Confronting our pain is not an easy process; writing can open us up, releasing our deepest selves to inform our lives. As John Fox has so beautifully demonstrated in his book *Poetic Medicine*, when a writer delves into raw emotion and experience to create a work of art, she is also doing the soul's work: making sense out of her life. Writing forces us to become keen observers of life, to pay attention and find the meaning in our experiences. We learn, out of our own self-confrontation and learning, to feel compassion for ourselves, for others, and for the world.

Lillian Baer reflected on the opening up to self and others that her cancer experience produced:

The Things We Love
By Lillian Baer

I love the gifts that my cancer experience has given me. I am more aware of life around me, and death, and in-between.

By having cancer, living through the treatments, I have slowed down the focus of my life. The saying "Stop to smell the roses" now has so much meaning. I have slowed down, smelling the flowers and seeing them too. With a clearer focus, it is like being able to taste an orange after having a stuffy nose. Like seeing the veins on a leaf drooping from a branch after tears have dried. A kiss has sensuality and also a texture, taste, and touch that is slow and in the moment.

So many gifts were mine as I came out of my first breast cancer experience, a new and special person in my life that would never before have been allowed in and so close. The awakening of taste buds and rose buds at different times and at the same time.

The gift of compassion: I feel more able to reach out to others in pain and suffering to a degree I only imagined before cancer became a part of me.

The gift of accompanying my brother during his final days with us, final breath, last sound and touch.

Gifts, and gratefulness.

Compassion, self-love, deepening, and awakening—surely this is part of the spiritual journey that we travel when we allow ourselves to write from our hearts, our lives, and our truths. Cancer writing, as Carolyn described so eloquently, can in this way become one's spiritual discipline, one's prayer book.

When Writing Is Spiritual

When we engage with our spirituality, we are quiet. Writing takes us into that quiet and allows us to find the center of ourselves. Writing is mindful, a meditation, a discipline. Spirituality also involves the practice of love, forgiveness, trust, and acceptance, and in writing and reading aloud together, we learn that we can be vulnerable. We learn to trust our own voices and ourselves. We learn that we can be loved and accepted for our truths and come to accept them ourselves. We learn to open our hearts to caring, to love, to our connectedness with one another. This is at the heart of our spirituality, and it is the heart of healing. The Irish poet Galway Kinnell wrote:

Sometimes it is necessary
to reteach a thing its loveliness
to put a hand on the brow of the flower
and retell it in words and in touch,
it is lovely,
until it flowers again from within,
of self-blessing.

Writing together is deeply affirming of one's own significance and beauty, of one's own humanity. "Someone wrote to me . . . that I was 'an inspiration,' Karen said, remarking on the valentines exchanged at the end of each series. "I used to feel so negative . . . and overwhelmed by it— fatigued, physically and emotionally taxed, and isolated from learning I could be myself. . . . I am able to be vulnerable with the writing group. I feel safe. I feel I can be seen—all that I feel I can say. I can be me."

The Importance of Ritual

Routine and ritual provide a sense of safety and security in the midst of a life turned upside down by cancer. When we write together, we treat our time with reverence and gratitude. We have learned to honor the importance of ritual as a way of inviting ourselves into community, into quiet and readiness to write. Our writing group rituals emerged naturally out of the shared group experience. They have become an integral part of our evenings together.

The Call to Writing

When we gather to write on Wednesday evenings, we greet each other with unmistakable fondness and appreciation for being together again. A buzz of greetings and conversation dominates the first few minutes of the evening. To signal our preparation to write, I light our "Circle of Friends" candle as an invitation to become quiet and enter the writing space.

Guided Imagery and Meditation

With the lighting of the candle, voices are stilled, and we settle into our places. I invite us to relax—closing our eyes if we wish, taking a few deep breaths to clear our minds—and then I begin with a guided imagery or meditation. The meditation allows us to center ourselves, acknowledge our gratitude to come together again, and become ready to write. I signal the end of the meditation by striking a small chime or Tibetan singing bowl, reading a selected poem or introducing an image as the context for the first writing exercise. The candle, the quiet relaxation, the meditation, and the chime have all become part of our weekly call to writing.

A "Singing" Chime

For the first ten weeks of the pilot program, I brought the timed writing exercises to an end with a verbal instruction, such as "You have one more minute" or "Bring it to a close." As much as I would do this gently, my verbal command seemed jolting and intrusive to the atmosphere of concentration and quiet. During the second series, I introduced the sound of a small Tibetan singing bowl or chime as our signal to enter the writing space and, at the conclusion of an exercise, I tapped the bowl again as a signal that it was time to stop writing. The beauty of the Tibetan chime was that it sang for several seconds after being struck, and we all liked the soft quality of the sound. The singing chime is now an integral part of our writing rituals.

Breaking Bread Together

It only took a few weeks before another aspect of ritual and celebration emerged. During the pilot program, I supplied snacks for our break each evening, most often nuts, brownies, and carrots or celery. As our group grew, so did the cost of the evening's refreshments, and very soon, I was exceeding my budget and digging deeper into my own pockets each week. One of the women offered a simple solution. "Let's all take turns," she said. Everyone agreed, and within two or three weeks, our modest snacks became a veritable feast. Two women share the responsibility at each meeting, and we eagerly anticipate our mid-evening break. Everyone looks forward to the surprises of each contribution: Homemade breads, brownies, salads, cheeses, and cookies adorn the small table at the back of the room.

During the break, I overhear the exchange of recipes, progress reports of treatments shared, and offers of help and support for those members who are experiencing particularly difficult times. Not only is food shared between us, but also the warm embrace of a supportive community, and our stomachs and spirits are full and nourished.

At the close of each series, we have a traditional potluck supper. No menu planning occurs. Every woman simply brings her own special dish, and again we share our stories, our food, our appreciation, and our affection for one another. Breaking bread together is deeply joyous and life affirming for all of us, and it has become an important aspect of shared community.

The Closing Circle

At the end of each evening, we always close with a poem, sometimes reading in unison, sometimes around the circle stanza by stanza or line by line. We linger over the beauty of the language for a few moments and the shared warmth of the evening before standing to join hands and form our closing circle. In these final few minutes of the evening I express gratitude for each woman's gifts of writing and offer our words of comfort and support to those in the group who are struggling through treatment, a recurrence, or some other difficulty. Our closing circle acts as an affirmation and acknowledgment of the bonds that have formed between the women, of the circle of friends who are traveling the cancer journey together.

The Gift of Valentines

Pat Schneider introduced the exchange of small written notes of appreciation for each writer in the workshop I first experienced with her at GTU in the summer of 2000. At the close of our week together, we wrote something memorable and appreciated about each other's writing on a three-by-five card, placing the cards in a small paper bag. It was so wonderfully affirming to take the small bag home, to read and reread the notes from each person. I quickly adopted this practice in my cancer writing groups, adding brightly colored envelopes and papers as I did. Our valentines are remembrances and acknowledgments of the beauty of one another's writing. It has become deeply important as a way of remembering our many weeks of writing together and sharing our stories and poems.

A Collection of Writing

At the conclusion of every ten-week series, we publish a collection of writing from the workshop. Originally entitled *Stories of the Journey,* it became the inspiration for this book. Our small publication is our remembrance of our ten weeks together, and it is the gift of our writing that we give to one another.

The criteria are simple. The women are invited to submit up to three of their pieces for each publication. Each must be something that was written in our time together, although some of the women refine or expand on the original piece after the workshop. I do not, for this publication, make substantial edits or changes to anything that is submitted to me. Because of the nature of our writing group, I believe that honoring the authentic and original writing each woman submits is more important than editing and refining it. Our publication is only distributed to the authors and to the library at the Community Breast Health Project.

Over the three and a half years that I have led the writing groups for the women at CBHP, I have seen the willingness to confront cancer strengthen, our writing deepen and grow. We have written touching portrayals of our cancer journeys. We have also written joyous stories of our healing, memories, and lives. Each issue of *Stories of the Journey* that we publish is a celebration of our ten weeks' together, a testimony to the courage of the women and to the healing power of writing and reading aloud together. The publication is eagerly awaited at the end of every ten-session series, and it is displayed in the CBHP library, available to other women who come to participate in the organization's many support programs. *Stories of the Journey* is a testimony to the resiliency of the human spirit and the courage of each woman in the struggle with cancer.

From Lament to Living

Early in the cancer journey, emotions run deep: bewilderment, disbelief, anger, and loss. I have observed that in the first few weeks of coming to terms with cancer, writing often takes the form of a lament, of grieving and loss. A diagnosis of cancer can feel like a betrayal from one's body, a loss of self after surgery or treatment, and the loss of breasts and hair. Almost any writing prompt elicits those raw, complex emotions during the first few weeks of writing together.

One evening, for example, I used abalone shells as the writing prompt, first giving each woman a shell to touch and feel as she sat with her eyes closed, then asking the women to examine the shell with their eyes open. Karen Jandorf examined the shell carefully and found that its shape reminded her of her lost breasts. She wrote:

Abalone Shell
By Karen Jandorf

I must have PMS.

I'm holding a shell—a breast-shaped shell—and that pisses me off.
Why couldn't I be holding a conch or a clam shell?
Why does the one I was given have to resemble a breast?
It even has a nipple, for God's sake!

Today I am angry.

Angry that I have no breasts.
Angry that reconstruction is such a detestable option to me.

Angry that I'm as flat as a table.
Angry that my breastbone hurts when I hug.
Angry that I used to like the feel of being naked and now can't
   dress fast enough.
Angry that I can't imagine ever making love again without a shirt
   on.

I'm angry.

Angry that I got a seashell shaped like a breast and not like a clam.

Unbelievable.
God, I hope I get my period soon!
Today I am angry.

I'm angry.

Karen's feelings of anger and loss are not uncommon, and in the beginning, it takes courage to share them aloud. But as these feelings of loss are shared with the group, we simply receive the writer's words and hold them as sacred, as gifts. Only unconditional acceptance and praise for specific elements of the writing are offered in response to reading. In this act of sharing, receiving and affirmation, we can move from lament to healing.

Lillian Baer was undergoing treatment for a recurrence of the cancer she had overcome just a year or so earlier. She questioned the meaning of having cancer a second time.

Talking to My Cancer
By Lillian Baer

Well, here we are—again. Are you the same as a few years ago? I know you are a different form, but you showed up in the same place in my other breast. Once again you dared me to take off my breast. Again, I refused, but that was arbitrary.

Why are you back? I know this is a test for me, an eye opener, another wake-up call, an encouragement, maybe even a gift. I can't really figure it out yet.

You have provided me the opportunity to try new things, ideas, activities, loves, movement, thoughts. Yes, you challenge me to be strong and also weak, to make decisions I never would have made before. You tease me with my life: should I fear you, fear death? Absolutely. Can we coexist? I suppose. Can I surpass, get the upper hand, come back again? We'll see.

You have allowed me a new look at my life, made me feel I want to run and do all the things I always put off.

Do I thank you or fear you, embrace you or just hold on for now?

On another evening, I presented the group with black-and-white photographs from the photographic essay *Winged Victory* by Art Myers. All the photos were of women who had undergone mastectomies. Karen Jandorf wrote again about her lost breasts, but in this poem, her anger and anguish had softened.

Winged Victory
By Karen Jandorf

You offer yourself . . .
your nakedness, your beauty.

Yes, your beauty.

Breastless and beautiful.
Flat and feminine.
Scarred and sacred, no longer scared.

Your eyes meet mine . . .
you reflect a future me.

You are a warrior spirit on an altar of light.

It occurs to me to wonder:
Did I wear my breasts as protection. . . ?
Did I lead with them to conceal what felt safer to hide?

Now that I no longer have that armor,
I must lead with my heart.

Someday I will light a candle,
create an altar of light and
offer myself as an Amazon Warrior.

Someday your eyes will meet mine . . .
my scars will be sacred,
my heart will be open and
I will say, "I am beautiful."

But until then,
thank you for showing the way.

The writing group serves as a community of support and love for these women, offering praise for surviving, for courage, for writing and telling one's story with honesty and authenticity. Each week I observe a gradual shift in emotions and in remembrances as the writing moves from grieving to thanksgiving: for life, for love, for the small gifts and blessings of each day, such as in the first part of Penny Warfield's short work, "Two Pieces":

Two Pieces
By Penny Warfield

I.

A light shines on my chronic disease like never before.
It has been twenty years since I was first diagnosed
but the light shines brighter now.
My 38-year-old daughter is pleading with me:
"Mom, you have to stay well—I need you to come stay with me
when I come home with my first child.
I have no idea what to do!"
For 20 years I have not worried about staying well.
But suddenly I am vulnerable.
A light is shining on my chronic disease:
my little girl needs me.

"Once I write about it," Jean said, "I can let go of the negative and embrace life. Sharing our experiences with this life-threatening illness has changed us. It is marvelous. It reconciles the fact that we are not just about cancer, but more than that. We bring memories to life. We write about life."

Surely this is the soul's work: coming face to face with our deepest selves, discovering our humanity, finding the meaning of our lives and, from that, a greater sense of love and compassion for the world. This is illustrated in Ceci's short piece, "The Cycle of Life":

The Cycle of Life
By Ceci Martinez

We travel a full circle in our life's journey here on earth. We start out helpless, needy, and dependent on others. And if we're fortunate to mature the full cycle, we once again become helpless, needy and dependent. Those of us who have shortened life spans will reach this stage sooner than others. I guess this is just nature's way of recycling—we start off crying as we emerge through our mother's womb, and later we return peacefully once again into the womb of God.

Witnessing and Being Witnessed

... my
jaws ache for release, for
words that will sway

anything. I force myself to remember
who I am, what I am, and
why I am here.
PHILIP LEVINE

Healing happens as we are heard. Writing and reading aloud to others is an act of witnessing—of self and of others. It has its roots in ancient religious traditions where confession and forgiveness were important rituals in spiritual life. In *Testimony: Crises of Witnessing in Literature, Psychoanalysis, and History,* authors Shoshana Felman and Dori Laub argue that personal recovery must include a conversation between the victim and a witness. This is also a basic tenet of psychotherapy and may explain why the act of writing and reading aloud together is so powerfully healing.

"If only we wrote without reading," Irena said, "it wouldn't be the definitive learning experience that it is. . . . We are together to give meaning to the life-altering disease we have been stricken with, to learn to integrate it into our lives. Listening and being heard is crucial."

"Every story," says Frank Ostaseki, who works with AIDS patients in San Francisco, "needs someone to listen."

As noted earlier, when we write, we often tap into painful memories and experiences. Writing enables us to reprocess our traumas. As we read aloud and are heard by others where our words are held as sacred, affirmed, and celebrated, we can hear ourselves and learn to accept ourselves fully. Not only are we our own witnesses to our lives as we share our work aloud; others also witness us. This is extraordinarily powerful and life-affirming. Writing together gives us the opportunity to discover the meaning of our individual experiences and integrate them into the fabric of our whole lives.

"It is as if," said one of my writers, "we each have a sermon, a sermon that we ourselves need to hear."

"It helps me find the meaning of my life—something of value that I can share," another writer commented. "If I can love your humanity," she said, "then I can love myself too. It ends the isolation."

"The only experience to which we can bear witness is that which we have personally endured or observed," Wallace Stegner wrote. In the writing group, each of us, leader and participant, knows intimately the experience of cancer and is uniquely equipped to bear witness to the others in the group. To bear witness is to offer support, to listen, to give another our complete attention, and to acknowledge the beauty and strength in her writing. Judy wrote:

> Surviving breast cancer is a journey that is as emotionally terrifying as it is physically challenging. . . . I've been able to explore my feelings within the warm and welcoming embrace of those who are making the same passage. I have been able to explore and share my hidden terrors, my hopes and joys with this compassionate group of women. With them, I have laughed and cried, vented frustrations, confronted my fears, and embarked upon the journey of healing.

When I asked the women to write a healing image for themselves one evening, Jean wrote a short poem she later titled "The Good Spell," explaining that her poem was informed by something she recalled from *The Good Spell Book*, instructing the reader to ask to be healed before going to bed. She read the poem aloud to us after writing it, made all the more poignant because we knew her valiant struggle and determination to overcome the aggressive cancer tumors that were spreading rapidly in her body.

The Good Spell

By Jean Allington

As I say the words,
"I want to be healed while I sleep,"
I breathe out with a sigh.
I imagine tiny, dark, cancer cells
floating out on my breath.

Out the window into the cold,
clear night. Rising, they crystallize
and sparkle, transforming,
floating up, rising together
forming bright new stars.

Rising to join the Pleiades
the birthplace of stars.
The Seven Sisters welcome these new beings
and become ten million strong.

Sending their bright blue light,
shining, illuminating my path
watching over me and blessing me,
the cells and I, each beginning a new life.

When I awake,
I will be miraculously recovered.
I worry a little though;
is the window open wide enough?

Varda, one of the group's most beloved writers, wrote with the Scribbling Women of CBHP for over two years before she lost her battle with metastatic cancer. She wrote about her cancer and her spiritual life.

Faith

By Varda Nowack Goldstein

God and I always had a special relationship, sealed in ancient Hebrew prayers and stained glass windows. The Shofar blown on Yom Kippur. The Book of Life open for ten days a year, and then my fate sealed.

But our relationship has changed. In asking me to surrender to this illness, God has asked me to let go—to trust—float free. And I have found this to be a most precious time.

My cancer has challenged my faith, and I have found an incredible well I did not know I had. I have found true surrender, enormous peace.

I have come home to God, and we have renewed our friendship.

A Picture of Varda

By Irena Olender

In this photograph you are still healthy or so it seems. You are wearing the white blouse with the silver blue stripes. It is a good complement to the color of your silver gray hair that has come in so thick, wavy and gorgeous after your recovery from chemotherapy. I am wearing the light blue sweater and deep blue vest that bring out the blue in my deep-set eyes. Your arm is around my shoulders. We are both smiling at the photographer and each other, our heads and bodies leaning into each other and joined together in a delicious meeting of the heart.

How does it happen, I wonder, that gradually, almost imperceptibly, a friendship unfolds and blossoms into sisterhood? It's hard to say, harder yet to catch the moment of the shift. In this picture that moment has already occurred. We are no longer just friends; we are sisters bound together in heart, soul, and spirit.

I remember the day this photograph was taken: a beautiful, warm weekday in January with clear, sunny skies, the best of California weather. The acacia trees were blooming in exuberant bursts of golden promises of abundant spring and life to come. You had taken time off from work to attend the special luncheon. Your wry, sardonic wit flashed in your animated description of your supervisor's dismay at your skipping out of an unexpected meeting. In a few lashing words you made her come to life from top to toe, inside and out. That's how you have always been: a sharp, intuitive observer, a master of words always skating on the thin edge of warmth, wit, and verbal warfare. It is easy to fly with you on the wings of that special talent. You and I are laughing, loving our bond of sisterly conspiracy. Suddenly the photographer comes around and snaps the picture.

I often look at this picture now, feeling the empty space left by your passing. I study it for signs, trying to remember you as you were then. It was the season of hope. You had decisively won the first round in your fight with breast cancer and everyone who knew and loved you shared in your optimism. Sure, you were still struggling with some problems in your eyesight, but those could be mostly attributed to the side effects of the chemotherapy. With the perfect clarity of hindsight I now wonder if those persistent symptoms might have been the first signs of the metastasis growing in your precious brain. Would it have made a difference, if we had noticed and understood sooner? It is highly unlikely, given the speed with which your illness progressed. There seemed to be no stopping it. Yet it is tempting to get lost in the possibilities of "if only" and "what if." It makes for an imaginary and temporary consolation for the grieving heart that seeks to undo the yet unacceptable. What a waste of time and energy! It is better to remember the way you show yourself to be in this picture, and the way you have always been: loving, warm, funny, creative, a friend and sister with incredible courage and impeccable integrity. Again and again I look at this picture. I see and remember you, and I am grateful.

My husband has put the photograph on the tansu, with sprigs of French lavender in an alabaster vase next to it. The milky, smooth texture of the alabaster matches your creamy, flawless skin. I see this picture, and I appreciate your beauty and spirit. I miss you, friend and sister. I miss you deeply. But I see and remember you, and I am grateful.

IO

The Valley of the Shadow of Death

You must grieve for this right now
—you have to feel this sorrow now—
for the world must be loved this much
if you're going to say "I lived."
NAZIM HIKMET

Earlier in this book, I wrote about my own discomfort in thinking of myself as a "survivor" of breast cancer. By the third series I was uncomfortable with the term, "breast cancer survivor" applied to anyone, although it is a commonly used term—even one I have used in the pages of this book. One potential new member had called at the beginning of the series to ask if the group was for survivors only. She was newly diagnosed and had not yet begun treatment. "I plan to be a survivor," she said, "but I don't think I could be called one yet."

I assured her the writing group was for any woman at any stage of the cancer journey. But the term "survivor" was also misleading in another way. For the second time in the life of the writing group, we were losing a member to metastatic cancer, a recurrence of her disease, although she had been truly a survivor for over two years.

During this time someone suggested, in an article that was passed by email from one "survivor" to another, that we dispense with the term "survivor," for it denoted victim mentality and obliterated one significant fact: all women who have suffered from breast cancer live to a greater or lesser extent with the possibility of recurrence. We were all women living with cancer and the knowledge that we can never again take life for granted, as Sheree's piece, "Just in Case," reminds us:

Just in Case
By Sheree Kirby

If I can see a cup drop to the floor and shatter, why can't I see it gather itself back together?

Sometimes, mostly in the middle of the night, I tell my husband that I'm scared. He asks me why. He tells me that I need to think more positively.

I'm not trying to think negatively, but the images that come to mind at the oddest of times frighten me. A funeral, friends saying nice things about me, my youngest daughter's tears.

Then I force an about-face, I imagine my white blood cells charging at the abnormal cells. I don't know if there are any abnormal cells left, but I have to imagine it anyway, just in case.

I'm doing a lot of things now, just in case.

I'm taking my supplements, just in case they help. I'm reading the latest, just in case there's information about a drug that might help women like me. I'm exercising daily, just in case it really does help keep my estrogen levels down. I'm thinking more positively, just in case my own mind can cure me. I ask those who are religious for prayers, just in case they work. I'm more present to the present, just in case that is all that I have.

Except when I am alone and tired, and I give in to the need to imagine a bleak future. Why is it easier to imagine such scenarios than to picture myself emerging strong and healthy? Is it some kind of premonition? Or am I preparing myself for the worst, just in case?

The Fear of Recurrence

The possibility of recurrence is always lurking in the shadows for women who have had breast cancer. The fear surrounding a recurrence made its way into the open one evening when, to stimulate the women's writing, I offered a photograph of one woman's hands reaching to another's. "Write about a time when someone reached out to help you," I said.

Marcia quickly moved to a smaller, adjoining room for privacy and began writing. She kept on writing a few minutes beyond the end of our timed exercise. When she rejoined the group, her face was flushed, her eyes moist with tears, yet she was smiling broadly. She volunteered to read aloud. We learned that in the two weeks between our group writing sessions, a sizeable lump had shown up in her one remaining breast. A second examination revealed more suspicious signs. Her doctor ordered more tests.

All the while, Marcia was showered with the love and support of her family and a group of women from her church who were part of her Bible study group. One of them accompanied her to the doctor's office for the third round of tests. Another delivered a basket of baked goods to her home while she was at the doctor's office. When Marcia's diagnosis was confirmed as a cyst, not a recurrence of breast cancer, she fairly danced from the doctor's office and was embraced enthusiastically by her friend. She read us the story of the ordeal and the supportive outreach from the circle of women.

We all sighed with relief when she neared her conclusion. We all understood the fear that had gripped her for those few long days between tests. We all experienced the elation of her reprieve. Women living with breast cancer—not just once in our lives, but harboring that niggling possibility that it could happen again.

Recurrence is the dark fear that we push as far from our minds as we possibly can. Women who have had breast cancer do survive it, yes, but we live with breast cancer in some form or another the rest of our lives. Our lives are forever altered by the experience. When I was diagnosed, an acquaintance called me to lend support. She had undergone a double mastectomy a year or so earlier. "You'll find that you've become part of a special sorority," she said. "You'll never be quite the same for this." I am still discovering what that means, and were it not for my own brief bout with the disease, I may never have found my way to leading my writing groups.

The women in my groups are all living with breast cancer. Many do survive and lead long and healthy lives; some do not, and a loss of a group member touches us deeply. Recurring cancers, debilitating side effects from treatments, and the possibility of metastases are all fears that lodge deep inside each woman who has ever suffered from this horrible disease.

When a Group Member Dies

Recall that our first experience of loss came early, just after our first pilot program. Wendy came to the group with metastasized cancer and the knowledge that she had only a few months left to live. As a physician, she spoke candidly about her illness and her prognosis. The rest of us still skirted around addressing our own fears of death and loss. Wendy taught us all to go there, name the fears, open them up, and face them. As I noted in an earlier chapter, I became a better writing group leader because of Wendy.

In the second year of the workshops, Carol, one of the original pilot program members, also suffered a recurrence. We were not prepared for Carol's diagnosis. She had finished her regimen of treatments only months before, dispensed with her wig in favor of a sporty short crop of dark hair, and returned to work. We had celebrated her victory. She had endured. She had survived. Now, less than a year later, the cancer showed up on her lungs. It had traveled from its original place and metastasized. More surgery and chemotherapy treatments were prescribed. She faced it squarely, exhibiting courage and the will to win her battle a second time.

During her second round of chemotherapy, Carol sent me an email, suggesting a writing exercise. "Why not have us write out the healing imagery we use to help ourselves deal with our fears or our treatments?"

she wrote. I answered immediately, telling her I would incorporate the exercise into our next writing session. I did, and this is what Carol wrote:

My Healing Imagery
By Carol Braunshausen

I am in the chair for chemotherapy. I see the clear plastic IV bag that holds the chemicals. My arm is outstretched, the needle in my elbow crease a straw ready to drink up the fluid. The bag is so full the seams are fairly bursting. The fluid is alive with floating bubbles of bright colors, small heart, butterflies. These are the prayers, the good wishes, the love that my friends have sent to support and nourish me.

The IV line has shape shifted. It is now a lightning bolt. It channels the bag's captured energy into my arm. I feel the cool progress through my veins. It curves at my shoulder and bursts into my chest, the heart of me. It courses through me, into the core of my being. It begins to spin, throwing off lights and colors like a fireworks ground display.

Sparks shoot from my fingertips, out of my eyes, through my pores. The particles suffuse me, pulsate through my every cell, cleansing and purifying, pushing out the cancer cells. Outside my body they are without power; they evaporate into nothingness. I glow with light that builds and brightens until it blurs the human figure in a crescendo of enormous energy radiating from my body.

The pulsing light begins to subside; it cools into pastel points that shimmer around me like a rainbow screen, an aura of love and caring that is tangible in its intensity. The colors settle on me like a shawl, wrap around me to reveal the form of the woman within. My body is clean and new and full of the love and prayers and energy that replaced the cancer space. I am lighter, radiant, and filled with something no longer visible that, in some mysterious way, can still be seen.

We were humbled by Carol's strength. We shared her hope; we shared her fears. And we worried. If Carol were absent from a session, one of us would call. "We missed you. Are you all right?" Gradually, driving to the workshop became difficult for her, so one of the members faithfully drove to Carol's house and brought her the twenty miles south to CBHP each Wednesday evening.

Just two weeks before the third workshop series ended, Carol's husband let me know she would not be returning to the group and that she was too weak to complete her submissions for our quarterly collection of the women's writing. I carried the news to the group, watching as some shed tears and others sat quietly, trying to quell their own fears. That night, we wrote "valentines" early for Carol, and I mailed them to her the next day. At the end of the series, we dedicated our publication of collected writings to her.

We prayed and hoped and waited, silently pleading for a miracle, but Carol's cancer steadily overtook her, and a few weeks later she died. Judy, who had become close to Carol in her final months, shared the experience of Carol's last days and the experience of the memorial service with the group. Carol's stories became part of her family's memorial and celebration of her life. Several were read aloud to family and friends at her service.

We mourned Carol's loss but were grateful for the time we had with her as part of our writing group. The gift in her loss was that it helped us to face our own fears of recurrence and death, and by coming together to grieve, we found comfort in each other and honored the life of one of our group members after her death.

Nevertheless, loss of a group member brings up our own fears of death from cancer. Judy wrote: "One of the hardest things is watching other women get sick and die. I wasn't ready to hear someone I'd been writing with was gone. How would I continue, knowing someone else would get sick and die? It brings my own mortality closer. It is the part of me that is holding my breath."

In the interviews he conducted for the PBS series *Healing and the*

Mind, Bill Moyers spoke with Dr. David Spiegel at Stanford Hospital about the impact of the loss of a group member in one of Spiegel's therapeutic cancer support groups. Spiegel remarked, "No doubt one part of what they were feeling was, 'There but for the grace of God go I.'"

"We are like a family now," Judy continued. "We know each other's heart and soul, what makes us laugh and cry. Carol was so strong, the last person you think would be conquered. It is terrifying when it is someone you really love but because of the writing experience, I had a secret knowledge and could hold her closer because of it."

Judy held Carol's memory close and kept vigil with her friend, giving her the chance to tell Carol what she meant to her before she was gone. I have found, in the work I have done leading bereavement support groups, that people often wish they could have had one more chance to tell a loved one how much she was loved or how much she is missed. It is no different for the women in our writing group. It is important to provide the opportunity to tell a dying member how much we care for her. When Wendy was in her last weeks, we each wrote letters to her. When Carol was no longer able to attend our sessions, we wrote her our "valentines," telling her what we loved about her writing and what she meant to each of us. These sessions were emotional but important ones for me, for they helped me realize that in a breast cancer writing group, or in any writing group where the experience of life-threatening illness is shared, we need to have a ritual to honor a lost member, allow us to get our grief and feelings into the open, and create the safety for us to express our own fears.

"As people face death," Marcia wrote, "it forces us to write about what we, too, are afraid of: to look death in the face. It is wonderful to be able to bring it into the open, let it be examined and felt so deeply." Responding to the poem, "Dawn Revisited," by Rita Dove, Marcia examined her fears of death:

Mortality

> *By Marcia Davis-Cannon*

We're different, we who have had cancer.
We can't saunter through life, unaware.
We confront our mortality early, and often.

Others may pretend they can live forever,
ignoring the finality of this existence,
but we know better.

Death wakes us in the night,
lodges between us and our partner in bed,
wriggles into the hugs we give our children.

We know we won't be here forever.
We don't know, can't know,
how long we have to live with that knowledge.

All we can do
is draw every delectable drop
out of every moment we have.

What would you do differently
if you knew you only had
the rest of your life to live?

Grieving together carries its own reassurances: we are not alone in this struggle. Sharing creates a much more observable closeness between group members. Grieving together affirms our lives. In the PBS interview, David Spiegel observed that grieving together gives "a message to us that when our time comes, we will not slip away unnoticed, but that we will be grieved and cared about and missed. . . . Seeing that what we do is appreciated and cherished by the people we care about makes dying less frightening than it otherwise would be."

The Scribbling Women suffered another loss just barely a year after Carol's death, and our sorrows ran deep. Varda, who had written in the group since the second series in 2001, began to complain of vision problems a year or so after ending her final round of chemotherapy. A medical examination in the summer of 2003 revealed a large brain tumor, and a biopsy confirmed that it was a metastasized cancer. For a few weeks, we took shelter in her extraordinary strength and our fervent hope for a miracle.

Varda was one of our most beloved writers, always finding the humor in life, despite all of its pain and struggle. Her only sister had died of metastatic cancer only two years earlier, and Varda had often written of their lives together as children. She wrote infrequently of her own cancer. "It has become who I am," she told me once, yet when she did choose to write about her cancer, her humor, courage, and honesty shone brilliantly in everything she shared. One evening, when I had asked the women to write about their scars, Varda used humor to soften the scars left behind by her breast cancer.

Scars

By Varda Nowack Goldstein

Vanity takes up a lot of time.

When I was younger, I was vain. Every morning I'd wake early and wash my long, black hair so that it would lie flat and straight to the middle of my back. I'd carefully cream my body and then exercise vigorously. I weighed myself every day and enjoyed admiring my tiny waist and flat stomach.

It's been a long time since I allotted hours of the day for primping. Age and cancer liberated me from my vanity.

After my first surgery to reduce my Double-D cups to a moderate size C, I was astounded by the intricate web of fine scars crisscrossing my breasts encircling the perimeters of each in bright red tissue. Within a year, I'd added the three scars from my stereotactic biopsies and then the large incision from my lumpectomy.

Infections after each surgery turned the drain exits into darkened mounds of scar tissue. Finally, a mastectomy and then emergency surgery to remove the infected implant turned my left side into a cat's claw design of scar upon scar, web upon web, circle within circle.

I am intrigued by my scar. I admire it. It has a pattern and a symmetry punctuated by three tiny purple radiation tattoos.

My scar ensures that I never take my cancer for granted. It is a living, breathing entity. Each day I spend an hour stretching and massaging the scar tissue to reverse the steady, relentless contraction of skin around muscle. Twice a week a therapist pulls and stretches the tissue; like the boy with his finger in the dike to hold back the water, he attempts to reduce my body's efforts to retract and protect my chest wall. The skin around the scar never really heals well. It remains sore and irritated—most of the muscle removed.

When I look at myself in the mirror, I find the scar fascinating, full of character and variation. My right breast seems somehow too plain, desperately lacking in charisma.

In the final months of her life, Varda came to the group to write, but not about her cancer, her fears, or illness. She wrote about her life, because life was the most precious thing to remember and capture in her stories. It was her legacy, and we delighted in sharing in her memories all that she had lived and become. She made us cry, and she made us laugh, creating unforgettable characters from her past, like her first date with the Bernstein brothers:

> In the fall of my freshman year, both Bernsteins asked me to the homecoming dance. My mother was positively gleeful. But how could I choose between twin brothers—twins I could barely tolerate?

I eventually accepted both dates. Harold picked me up, handed me a lovely wrist corsage, and escorted me to dinner. After dinner, Herbert joined me at the entrance to the dance floor. He also brought me a corsage that I pinned to the bodice of my very revealing gown.

I had a surprisingly enjoyable evening and found that a legend builds up around a girl with two corsages, two dates and a great pair of breasts. And much to my mother's delight, I was never without a date on weekends.

In August 2003, Varda underwent another surgery, this time to remove the brain tumor. We all knew the prognosis. With an aching heart, I convened a special session of the writing group: an evening to write, I told the women, in honor of Varda. Everyone came that evening, even former writing group members. We crowded into the small living room at CBHP, waiting for Varda's arrival.

A short time later, the door opened, and Irena led her friend Varda—still unsteady on her feet, supported by a walker—into the room. The women crowded around her, welcoming her with smiles, tears, and long and affectionate embraces. That night, all the Scribbling Women celebrated Varda's life and her presence in the writing group. We wrote our love and our prayers for her. We read aloud. We wept, and we laughed together as Varda regaled us with another of her wonderful stories from her childhood in New York City. We feasted on fruits, cheeses, breads, and desserts that the women brought. We gathered around Varda at the closing and offered her our love, reciting together a Navajo night chant, "Happily may I walk," but changing the words from "me" to "you" as an offering of our love for Varda.

> Happily may you walk.
> May it be beautiful before you.
> May it be beautiful behind you.
> May it be beautiful below you.

May it be beautiful above you.
May it be beautiful all around you.
In beauty it is finished.

That August evening was the last time Varda wrote with the Scribbling Women of CBHP, an evening that will forever remain in our hearts and minds. A few weeks later, Varda slipped into a coma, and on the eve of Rosh Hashanah, her family stood vigil as she quietly passed away.

After her death, we wrote our remembrances. For weeks, we felt her presence in the group. In my letter to Varda as my remembrance of her, I wrote: "A week after you died, I held a writing workshop in my home. I shuddered when a new writer sat in the wine-colored leather chair that you always took as yours. For a moment, I expected to hear you squeal, 'Ouch! I'm sitting here,' so palpable was your presence."

Another friend, Carolyn, wrote a poem, "Elegy," mourning her death and honoring their different religious heritages of Catholicism and Judaism.

Elegy
By Carolyn Schuk

Varda, in your wedding picture
A girl with luminous sable hair and a lambent smile
Shared hopeful cake. Now in place of that generous mantle
Gray fledgling down covers relentless scars marking
Battle lines drawn and redrawn: Varda fought here.

I touch your hand under the blanket, regrets
Flock like migrating birds around me—
They perch on my outstretched arm: How I wish
We had been young together just starting out
In that hopeful universe

That is always the patrimony of youth. How I wish
We were mothers together—
Young and hip, never square soccer moms in sweatpants and vans.
But wishes are done.

You once wrote
In the picture there is a happy family,
That picture is a lie.
Who will speak such truths now you are gone from us?

You breathe, now labored, now peaceful. You stir.
I do not know if you hear me as I say,
Varda, it's Carolyn. Varda, I love you.

Ye vor rak Adonai v'yish meh reh chor
Keyne Yehe ror Sion

Requiem aeternum
dona eis domine
et lux perpetua luceat eis.

Ya air Adonai p'nav aileh chor
Layne Yehe ror Sion

Agnus dei qui tollis
peccata mundi
dona eis requiem
sempiternam

Ye sa Adonai p'nav aileh chor
V'yeh same
Le cha shalom
Kayne Yehe ror Sion.

Requiem aeternum dona
eis Dominie
et lux perpetua luceat eis

Requiescat in pace
Rest in sacred time
Rest in time without end
Rest.

After Loss: The Legacy of Story

We wanted to give Varda's family a gift of remembrance. A few weeks after her death, I bound the women's letters to her together with a collection of her writings that had been published in our booklet of collected writing, and titled it *Varda, A Writer Remembered*. The first section contained the women's letters to Varda, and the second section contained all of Varda's published pieces from her two years in the writing group. This was our greatest gift to Varda's family, a small remembrance of her life through her stories.

Varda's husband called me the night he received the booklet, speaking haltingly through his tears, overcome with emotion, yet grateful. "I couldn't put it down," he said. "You have no idea what it means." Perhaps I didn't, at least not completely, but I was beginning to realize that the power of writing to heal extended well beyond the individual women in the writing group. It touched the lives of their loved ones. Their poems and stories were testimony to their lives, a legacy to be read and shared again and again. Several days later, Varda's husband called again. "May I copy this and send it to her relatives and friends? It would mean so much to them."

"Yes, of course," I said. I knew for certain that Varda would be remembered through her stories for a long time to come. A few weeks later, Varda's daughter, Lusana, wrote her thank-you in a touching letter to the women in the writing group, reminding us again of the power of story to keep alive the legacy of a loved one's life. As I read Lusana's letter, I knew for certain that the healing power of writing together had extended well beyond the confines of the writing group.

It's a cool Texas afternoon when I receive a white parcel containing a book written by the Scribbling Women and dedicated to my mom, Varda Goldstein. . . . With my legs tucked underneath me I sit on the living room couch and immediately begin poring over the book's contents. It is here on my couch, with my children playing near my feet, that I begin to imagine the women putting their memories to paper. Brave women, strong women, scared women, and women disheartened by the loss of one of their own, a friend and fellow writer. . . . I do not stop reading. Not to answer the phone or begin doing any of the many household chores that are calling me. I just read. I read, and I weep, overwhelmed by emotion.

"What's wrong, Mommy?" my two-year-old child asks me with a look of genuine concern on his tiny, cherubic face.

"Mommy is just thinking about Grammie," I say, assuring him and myself that I am fine. That everything is going to be all right. Everything is going to be all right. I know this. In my head I know this. The sun will continue to rise and set each day and night. . . . And memories of my mom will continue to play in my mind, reminding me daily of how precious life is. I know now that everything will be all right. . . .

To the Scribbling Women: thank you for your memories, another piece to remember my mom by. You will always be in my thoughts and prayers.

Cancer as a Part of Our Lives

"Aren't you done with that yet?" the husband of one group member asked as she signed on for another writing group session. She told the story to us one evening and shook her head. "He doesn't understand about that part," she said. And yet, the original impetus to write ourselves through cancer shifts. Cancer becomes part of the fabric of our life experience, and while always present, it recedes from prominence. Cancer, Alice Hoffman wrote, is not the whole life, only a chapter.

During this passage from pain into possibility, from wounding into healing, the joy of writing takes hold and we take pleasure in telling the stories of our lives. There is healing, and in the healing, there is laughter and joyousness: first loves, first dates, first bicycles, chocolate, memories of parents, relatives, school, teachers, nature, love, children. Life. Lives fully experienced and lived.

"Having a life," as Susan Sontag said, "is about tragedy and sorrow as much as it is about joy and contentment." Writing honors the human experience in a way that perhaps nothing else can do. And night after night, as I write with the women in my breast cancer groups, I am reminded of the richness of life: the gifts of story; the courage, the fears, the self-doubts; the deep, shared intimacy of opening up our emotions and our lives to one another in safety; the release, letting go, the healing. And I am certain my work, my vocation, makes a difference in others' lives. For what greater gift could I ask?

Breakfast Lesson
By Sharon Bray

An over-ripe banana
lies here on my plate.
Speckled brown age spots
on its pale yellow skin—
an older banana.

An aging woman,
eyeing her face in the mirror,
sees the appearance of tell-tale brownish splotches,
applies the spot fading cream
purchased from the cosmetics counter
in a moment of vanity.

I peel back the skin of the banana.
Inside, its smooth creamy flesh
is unblemished, soft and luscious.
Beauty, my mother once told me,
is more than skin deep.

II

On Being a Writing Group Leader

I'm just a guy, thirty-eight years old, who had a
heart attack. I'm okay now, but I learned a lot.
Fleischmann's margarine commercial, 1986

Earlier, I mentioned that I first began my cancer writing group just a few months after I took Pat Schneider's workshop at the Graduate Theological Union in Berkeley. Whether it was a sense of excitement and urgency that propelled me forward or many years of teaching, group facilitation, and counseling adults that gave me the confidence to try, I cannot be certain. Yet the complexity of being a writing group leader with women who have cancer continues to be revealed to me in many small ways each time we meet and write together.

What qualities, I wondered, did the writers believe were important in the leader? I decided to ask them. It might seem a little like expecting a leader to leap tall buildings at a single bound, but here are some of their responses:

Being a breast cancer survivor and a writer with true compassion, strong interior stability and good management skills.

Holding the space without coloring the field; knowing that she is key to the process but not central to it;

reflecting back what seems to be the essence of the piece; meeting the writer where she is . . . Understanding of group process and dynamics . . . and if the workshop is focused on healing or recovery, some experience in or exposure to a helping profession and understanding of what people are healing or recovering from.

Being a writer herself; being a survivor; having some psychological training or leadership background to lend depth and insight.

Patience, engendering trust, group work skills, sensitivity, reliability, predictability, and compassion.

Supportive, supportive, supportive.

Affirming. Able to create a safe environment and encourage the writer no matter where her skills are.

Positive and encouraging, and treats everyone with respect and equal importance.

Loving acceptance of the participants; a sense of humor; willingness to share herself and her work; discrimination and firmness; sincerity.

A compassionate and caring nature; empathy and a sympathetic spirit; a positive attitude; a great sense of humor; concern, respect, and consideration.

The Necessity of Experience

What mix of qualities and experience do I think are important in leading healing writing groups?

Experience with Life-Threatening Illness and Loss

Does one have to be a woman who has had cancer to lead a group of breast cancer survivors? I don't think it is a prerequisite, but it can help, at least in the beginning. Cancer is the common bond between us, and even though I feel my own experience was lightweight in comparison to most of the women in the groups, we all began with a common language and understanding. Facing down a life-threatening illness changes one's life in deep and discernible ways. Any direct experience with terminal or life-threatening illness, loss, and bereavement would serve to inform the prospective leader who wishes to lead a writing group for individuals diagnosed with cancer or other life-threatening illness. However, the experience of having had cancer or another life-threatening illness is not, of itself, enough to enable one to become a writing group leader.

Knowledge from the Helping Professions

The Amherst Writers & Artists method carries with it certain fundamental practices for its participants, and the intensive training is invaluable for any aspiring workshop leader as a way to keep the writing group about writing, not about therapy. Yet, in the context of the breast cancer survivors' group, I have felt the benefit of my other background and training time and time again—skills in counseling, group work, and teaching. My background has helped to inform my role as a group leader, especially in my writing groups for women living with cancer.

My own experience suggests that if one seeks to lead a "healing" writing group like the breast cancer groups, it may help to have some exposure or prior experience with the helping professions, though it is not necessarily a requirement. So much depends on the depth and maturity of the person. However, in these kinds of groups, the line between a healing writing group and a therapy group is very thin. The prospective leader needs a genuine understanding of the boundaries between therapy and writing, must be able to appreciate those boundaries and be able to maintain them.

Keeping Your Own Ego at Bay

A critical practice of the AWA method is that the group leader writes and reads with the group, being just as authentic and vulnerable in her writing as she is asking her participants to be. I have found that, as leader, I am never able to go as deeply into my own writing as the other women. Nor am I, a former thespian, able to "perform" my written work with as much expression as I might like to do. I have one eye on the clock; another, from moment to moment, on the women. Sometimes I don't read at all, because it is most important to give every woman a chance to read and be affirmed. Other times, I read something that I know is not as good as I would like, but I do it to help lessen the anxiety that some of my more reluctant readers may have. More than once, I have counseled a prospective workshop leader in my sessions: "If you want to lead a writing group, then you need to take your performer backstage."

Knowing When; Knowing How

The emotions that are expressed in our writing groups are powerful and poignant. Sometimes I fight off the urge to rush to the woman who has just read and throw my arms around her, saying, "There, there . . . it will be all right." Instead, as the AWA method teaches, I hold the writer's words gently and reverently, and focus on the beauty of the language, the courage she demonstrates to write so honestly, and the writing. I maintain the safety for the writer to open up and express all that she thinks and feels about her cancer journey in doing so.

I pay attention to the delicate shifts, the silences, the body language, the feedback of the other women, modeling when I can, gently correcting someone when they lose sight of the line between affirming and interpreting, and sometimes making a mental note of someone who might need other kinds of help. I pray, most evenings, before I begin, asking for guidance and an open heart as I lead the writing exercises.

Keeping the Group Healthy and Open

The writing groups I lead for women living with cancer are offered through community organizations. In my larger community, I work with the Community Breast Health Project and the Bay Area Breast Cancer Network, nonprofit organizations that offer free programs and services to women diagnosed with breast cancer. As a community service, it is important for the writing group to stay true to its raison d'être: helping women through their cancer journey through writing. Writing together is joyous and affirming, and it creates a strong social community among the women.

As the writing program continued to gain more attention from women who sought the supportive services through CBHP, so did our realization that the group was inadvertently becoming "closed" to newcomers, with a solid core of long-term regulars who were coming together to write, their cancer experiences well behind them. New members sometimes felt uncomfortable or intimidated by the close community and the writing of the long-term members. We were in danger of eroding the underlying reason for the writing program and, in doing so, the health of the writing group. I talked frankly with the regulars, and with the support of CBHP, created a short-term "transitional" writing group for them, focusing more on developing craft and encouraging them on to other writing experiences outside CBHP.

In the ongoing series, I now offer women the opportunity to write together for three consecutive series before going on the waiting list to make room for newcomers. And of course, if any of the women suffers a recurrence, they are welcomed back into the writing group at any time. It was a happy complication to have the writing program become so popular, but it was also a learning opportunity for how, at the very beginning of each new series, to set and manage expectations for writing together.

Love and Appreciation of Writing as Art and Craft

"I don't care about writing and publishing," a new workshop leader told me. "I just care about leading healing writing groups." It is hard to imagine not caring about writing if one wants to lead a creative writing group, whether it is to help individuals heal from traumatic life events or simply to discover the power of their voices through writing. It is not necessary to have an eye toward publishing in order to lead a writing group like the ones for women living with cancer, but I fervently believe a leader has to love to write, read, continually expand, and deepen her own writing to be a writing group leader. I find the desire to want only to lead "healing" writing groups unsettling, no matter how well intended, if it is not coupled with a driving passion for the art and craft of writing. Without that passion, we may cross over the line between leading creative writing groups that also are healing, as the ones I describe in this book, and therapy groups that also write. It is, in the context of the groups I lead for women living with cancer, a fine line, but necessary. In AWA method writing groups, healing happens through writing together in a supportive group, not from intervention or interpretation of our writing by a therapist.

Humility and the Willingness to Learn

It is part art form perhaps, but deeply grounded in all the experience I have had as a counselor, a group leader, a teacher, and a writer. I am continually humbled by the courage, strength, and gifts of each woman in my cancer writing groups. I continue to learn from each woman in every session I lead. The willingness to learn from others is a necessary part of being a writing group leader.

The Willingness to Learn

I came to understand the importance of self-awareness and the desire to continually learn several years ago when I conducted my doctoral research in the School for Landscape Architecture at the University of Guelph. I was investigating the way instructors think during teaching, and I was especially interested in the role of critical self-reflection—the use of one's experience—in facilitating the growth of expertise. Ron, one of the youngest members of the faculty, was also one of the most highly regarded instructors. Despite the praise he routinely received from his students, he was humble and naturally curious about teaching, constantly eager to improve his own teaching skills. Of all the instructors I studied, Ron was the only one who consistently reflected on his own teaching, seeking feedback and acting on it consciously to improve his classroom skills. It was no surprise to me when, just a few years later, Ron won a prestigious 3M teaching award. After I completed my dissertation, he wrote a short letter to me, entitled "The White Rat Talks Back." In it, he described his journey of learning and growth in the classroom, the pain of making mistakes, of being observed by another, and his struggle to learn better skills. He ended the paper with a quotation from a Fleischmann's margarine commercial that I have never forgotten: "I'm just a guy, thirty-eight years old, who had a heart attack. I'm okay now, but I learned a lot."

I'm OK Now, But I've Learned a Lot

"Writing," Warren Bennis wrote in *On Becoming a Leader*, "is the most profound way of codifying your thoughts, the best way of learning from yourself who you are and what you believe." Writing this book has forced me to reflect on and articulate what has informed my own work. I have learned a lot from my own cancer journey and from the Scribbling Women of CBHP. I have learned that no matter how small one's experience with cancer is, it changes you forever. I have learned that it is not enough to simply want to help others to heal—although the desire will take you much closer to doing the work. I have learned to be fully present for each woman in a way I never was able to before. I have learned to listen without judgment and to find the beauty in each woman's words. I have learned when to let the silence linger after someone reads and when to move quickly into it when a writer has been especially vulnerable. I have learned to be in the presence of illness and of death, and not to shrink from its reality. I have learned that, in order to heal and be healing to others, I have had to suffer, to struggle with my own darkness, to fail and to overcome hardship. I have learned from the courage, compassion, and enormous strength of human spirit of these women. I am learning, above all else, what it truly is to be human.

Leading the healing writing groups with breast cancer survivors is joyous work. Weekly I receive the gifts of their stories, prose and poetry. I watch them enter, wounded and in distress from their diagnoses and treatment, and as the weeks go by, gain in strength and self-empowerment. I hear their voices grow stronger, deeper, and more lyrical and beautiful. I hear them claim themselves as artists, as writers. And I watch them receive and give the gifts of affirmation and love to one another. It is the most deeply important work I have ever done.

Healing through Writing: Some Final Comments

This has been our healing journey as women living with cancer: writing and telling our stories through the experience of cancer helped us move on with our lives. When our stories were shared, the interpersonal connections that formed gave us the safety and the support to reflect on all that our lives had been—and all that we had become. Not only did writing and sharing our stories help us process the intense and stressful aspects of breast cancer, but it provided a sense of renewal and relief, satisfaction and joy. Writing together has been life giving for many of us. For others, writing provided solace and support in the final months of life. Writing together provided a way to honor those women whose disease overtook them. It gave them the opportunity to leave us their legacies through their stories and poems. We reaffirmed the universality of our life experiences as we wrote and shared our stories, and yet, we also affirmed and heard the uniqueness of our individual gifts. Writing and sharing our stories gave voice to our humanity and to our capacity for creation. And we remembered and honored how very precious life is.

Just a few weeks ago, Jean described her gratitude for the writing group as she wrote from her hospital bed, undergoing further treatments to combat the metastases in her body. Perhaps she says it best for all of us:

> Scribbling Women helped me find my long hidden voice and
> . . . to sing again. Without Scribbling Women, I would have buried
> my sorrow, my pain. I would be dead by now. The encouragement

and love that enfolds me each week and in between sessions, the warmth and kindness, the gifts that are given me, brought out of the darkness of a surely terminal diagnosis, have made me believe that I will survive this, and much more.

This is testimony to all we experienced. This is the healing power of writing together through cancer.

Starting Here, What Do You Want to Remember?
By Kathy Walters

A gathering of women—
discovering themselves
sharing those discoveries
delighting in each other's stories
caring for one another

Starting here, what do you want to remember?

Vibrant women—Wendy, Carol, Varda
The privilege of sharing in their lives
The privilege of sharing in their deaths

Starting here, what do you want to remember?

Truth
Beauty
Courage
Laughter

Starting here, what do you want to remember?

The magic
The power
The communion
The love

EPILOGUE

It is early spring in Menlo Park, California, and the trees are already coming into bloom. Springtime is always a time of hope, new life, and of new possibilities for me. Nearly four years ago, breast cancer came to me in the springtime. Whether I knew it then or not, cancer gave me an entry into a new life. As I think back on the past four years, I am conscious of the different skin I wear as a result of those unexplainable life forces that drove me back to writing during the summer of 2000 and, a few months later, into conceiving and offering the first writing group to women who were diagnosed with breast cancer. Since then, my work has expanded and deepened, and through the writing groups, I have fulfilled my search for joyous, meaningful work.

Jean, one of our regular writing group members, has just been admitted to the hospital this past week. They've found metastases on her vertebrae. We are unsure of her prognosis. Her spirit and courage humble us as she continues to undergo even more tests, and our hearts are heavy. Yet the entire writing group has mobilized, adding to the circle of supportive friends and family who surround her already. We supply her with cards, calls, visits, and volunteer help, ensuring her day-to-day needs are met and that she knows the strength of our love and prayers for her victory over this disease.

Last night, I spoke with Jean by telephone, and she told me how much she missed attending the writing group. I know how very important Jean's writing has become in her struggle with cancer. Last summer, when she began an experimental drug program to inhibit the growth of her tumors, I gave her a small leather-bound journal to write in during the many weeks of treatment. She has carried it into our Wednesday sessions ever since, and she continues to fill its pages with poems and stories of her life and her struggle with cancer. During our telephone conversation last night, Jean told me she'd asked one of the women to bring her the writing prompts she would miss each week while she is hospitalized. "I'll do better than that," I told her, "I'll send you a list of thirty or forty of my best writing prompts so you can use them to write as much as you want." I hung up the receiver and printed out a long list of writing exercises and sent them to her. I had tears in my eyes the entire time.

It is difficult to imagine what life was like before my own experience with cancer. My world was rearranged in those many months, and in writing and leading writing groups for cancer survivors, I have never looked back with regret. Now, it is hard to imagine life without the extraordinary gifts of love and compassion I witness each evening when our writing groups convene, hard to imagine a week that passes when I am not reminded of just how precious life is, and how, in our relentless and driven world, we sometimes lose ourselves so completely, feeling alone and isolated.

It is the community of women living with cancer who ground me and reaffirm that my work has meaning. It is this same group of women who, as they come together to share the stories of their lives, remind me of our common humanity and connectedness to a world much larger than ourselves. And it is that same community of women who have helped me to deepen my own life, my spirituality, and my gratitude for the joy of doing this work. Now, I cannot imagine my life without leading writing groups with women who struggle so valiantly with cancer. This book is as much theirs as it is mine.

Selected Writing Exercises

In her book *Writing Alone and with Others,* Pat Schneider has included many of her original and time-tested writing exercises as well as several dozen "new" exercises gathered from her network of Amherst Writers & Artists' affiliates and alumni. Pat's book is an invaluable resource for every writing group leader, and when I first began leading my breast cancer survivors' writing groups, I relied heavily on the prompts I had experienced in the first AWA training.

However, I was eager to build up my collection of writing prompts. Soon my bookshelves were filled with books about writing, my file drawers fairly bursting with ideas and exercises, and I tried several new prompts in each ten-week workshop series. Some were more successful than others; some worked well for one group of women and not as well for a later group. Gradually, I have built a repertoire of many different writing exercises, and I continue to try new ones.

Nearly any writing prompt can take the writer to the memory or emotions that beg to come out into the open. This has been confirmed over and over in my work with breast cancer survivors as well as in bereavement groups or with at-risk teens or older adults. Nevertheless, I have also modified or developed a number of exercises to specifically address the experience of cancer. I have included several of those exercises that have been particularly powerful for women living with breast cancer. Whether writing together in a group or writing alone in one's journal, these exercises are ones I've found especially evocative in writing about one's journey through cancer.

1. **Fear:** Raymond Carver's poem "Fear" is an excellent stimulus to invite an individual to address the terror, darkness, and gut-wrenching fear that cancer can provoke. I provide each person a copy of the poem, inviting one of the members to read it aloud. Sometimes I will also read it aloud a second time before inviting them to write about their fears, beginning with the line "fear of," as in Carver's poem. Have a box of tissues available.

2. **Cancer Words:** Ask each group member to take three or four minutes to list as many cancer-related words as they can. Then, as a group, take a few minutes to call out the words to one another. Invite the group members to add to their list when they hear words that particularly resonate with their experience. Now, invite them to write, using any of the words to take them into their memory or experience of cancer.

3. **Diagnosis:** Use Chia Martin's poem "Diagnosis," Raymond Carver's "What the Doctor Said," or "Snapshot of a Lump" by Kelli Agodon to introduce the exercise. Read the poem aloud together, then invite the participants to begin writing with the line, "When the doctor said . . ."

4. **Hair:** Lucille Clifton's poem "Hair" always evokes smiles and laughter and serves as a stimulating prompt to the group to write about hair—having it and losing it.

5. **Look in the Mirror:** I pass around a hand mirror to the group members, inviting them to take a look at the image of themselves reflected back. Then, I have the group members close their eyes and imagine themselves as they were before cancer. How have they changed? How has their life been altered? "What feelings do you notice as you look back at the person you were before cancer?" I let them linger with the imagery for a few moments, then invite them, when they are ready, to begin writing.

6. **Scars:** I use a number of different poems about scars, for example, those written by Chia Martin, Marilyn Hacker, Lucille Clifton, or Joe Milosch, among others. Our scars tell many stories of our lives. Think about the scars on your body, whether they are visible or not. Choose one of your scars. Tell its story.

7. **Gratitude:** As the women in my breast cancer group end treatment and begin to reconstruct their bodies and their lives, I often see a shift toward hope and making plans for the future. Most have overcome extraordinary odds or excruciating treatment regimens. In this exercise, I have used an Iroquois prayer of Thanksgiving, excerpts from Audrey Lorde's cancer journals, or Alice Hoffman's *New York Times* article about her cancer experience as an introduction. Then I simply invite them to write about those things for which they are grateful.

8. **A Gift for Myself:** Being kind to ourselves during the experience of cancer is harder than one might imagine. The complexity of emotions, anger, recriminations, and "should be" can be heard from nearly everyone. In this exercise, I invite some self-tenderness. I pass around a small gift-wrapped package as I ask the question, "If you could give yourself one gift today, what would it be?"

9. **Cancer Metaphors:** Language is a powerful mechanism for shaping our thoughts and actions. As we begin this writing exercise, we talk about imagery and metaphors that shape our lives. I ask them: What are the messages we give to ourselves in the images we choose to describe our lives? How do you think of your cancer? A journey? A crisis? A battle? I invite the participants to explore the metaphors and images they hold about their cancer experience and write about them.

10. **Talking Back to Cancer:** In this exercise, we bring cancer right into the open and give it a voice, a persona. I invite the group members to imagine themselves facing their cancer, eyeball to eyeball, and talking back to it. Talk back to your cancer, I say, as I invite them to write.

11. **Head Turners:** In this exercise, the stimulus is a number of photographs of women without hair, all undergoing chemotherapy. We were fortunate, the first time we did this exercise, to have access to a book-in-

progress that featured women without hair and their stories. I invite the women to look at the photographs and then to write about the beauty, the strength, and the courage of the women pictured, and of themselves.

12. **Helping Hands:** Having cancer is a time when we can experience the love and caring of friends and family as never before. Sometimes people reach out to us in ways we never expected, and we are touched by their compassion and concern. In this exercise I pass around a photograph of one woman's hands reaching to another's. I suggest simply that they think of a time in their cancer journey when someone reached out to them. It might have been a family member, a prayer group, colleagues at work, a neighbor, or someone quite unexpected.

13. **Winged Victory:** I found in a used bookstore a copy of the beautiful photographic essay *Winged Victory*. Each page was a photograph of a woman who had undergone a mastectomy, and the photographs were extraordinarily beautiful. I placed them on a long table and invited the women to look at each photograph, and then write. The writing was deep, poignant, and enormously powerful. It is now part of my regular repertoire with new breast cancer writing groups.

14. **The Rest of Your Life:** This exercise began as a result of another poem, "Dawn Revisited" by Rita Dove, that I'd read aloud to the women, inviting them to focus on the line, "Imagine you wake up with a second chance. . . ." Again, the writing was beautiful and evocative of the journey. One writer, Marcia, ended her poem with "Imagine you wake up and have the rest of your life to live." That has now become a writing prompt for the women. I introduce it through a short guided imagery, having them imagine how they would like their lives to be, concluding with the quote from Marcia's poem.

15. **Our Spiritual Images:** I borrowed this exercise from John Fox's *Poetic Medicine*. Fox describes poems as vessels for the soul, but also as full of story and emotion, captured in powerful images and metaphors. I invite the women to think about their own sacred symbols they carry within themselves, such as a dove, moon, star, eagle, or cross, for example. Then I suggest they begin writing, including the symbol or image in the opening line "I am a _____" and write.

16. **Writing Your Healing Imagery:** This wonderful exercise came from Carol Braunshausen, one of our group members who died from metastatic cancer in 2002. Carol had been using a healing imagery to help her deal with her regimen of chemotherapy. One night, she suggested we write our healing images and read them aloud to one another. The writing was vivid, descriptive, and powerful. I have also used a variation of this, which uses a garden as the prompt. I invite the women to imagine a healing garden and describe it.

17. **A Letter to Myself:** Writing directly to someone can induce powerful emotions and prose. It can also be a way to address ourselves: the ones we were in the past, the ones we are now or wish to be. Invite the women to write a letter to themselves before cancer, or to the self they have become with cancer.

18. **Asking the Hard Questions—Life and Death:** Three poems have proved to be particularly powerful writing prompts with the women in my breast cancer groups. One, "Questions in the Mind of the Poet as She Washes the Floors," by Elena Georgiou, has opened up the women's writing by taking them directly into the "big" life questions we all share. The other, "I Will Not Die an Unlived Life," by Dawna Markova, confronts our fear of mortality and our determination to live a full and meaningful life for the time we have left on earth. The third, "Things I Didn't Know I Loved," by Nazim Hikmet, also elicits wonderful writing.

REFERENCES AND RESOURCES

Adams, Kathleen. *Journal to the Self*. New York: Warner Books, 1990.

Albert, Susan W. *Writing from Life: A Guide to Telling the Soul's Story for Women on an Inward Way*. New York: J. P. Tarcher/Putnam, 1997.

Anderson, Charles M., and Marion M. MacCurdy, eds. *Writing and Healing: Toward an Informed Practice*. Urbana, Ill.: The National Council of Teachers of English, 2000.

Baldwin, Christina. *Life's Companion: Journal Writing as a Spiritual Quest*. New York: Bantam Books, 1991.

Bennis, Warren G. *On Becoming a Leader*. New York: Perseus Books, 2003.

Berman, Jeffrey. *Risky Writing: Self-Disclosure and Self-Transformation in the Classroom*. Amherst: University of Massachusetts Press, 2001.

Bolton, Gillie. *Reflective Practice: Writing and Professional Development*. London: Paul Chapman Publishing, Ltd., 2001.

————. *The Therapeutic Potential of Creative Writing: Writing Myself*. London: Jessica Kingsley Publishers, 1999.

Bray, Sharon A. "The Scribbling Women of CBHP." *The CBHP Report*, December 2001.

Broyard, Anatole. *Intoxicated by My Illness*. New York: Ballantine Books, 1992.

Buford, Bill. "What Is Narrative Anyway? Part III: How We Tell Stories." In Chip Scanlan, *Poynteronline*, October 7, 2003.

Cameron, Julia. *The Artist's Way: A Spiritual Path to Higher Creativity.* New York: J. P. Tarcher/Putnam, 1992.

Cancer as a Turning Point: From Surviving to Thriving (audiotapes). Boulder, Colo.: Sounds True Publishers, 2000.

Carver, Raymond. *All of Us.* New York: Vintage Books. 2000.

Charon, Rita. "Narrative and Medicine." *The New England Journal of Medicine* 350, no. 9 (2004): 862–64.

Clifton, Lucille. *The Terrible Stories.* Rochester, N.Y.: BOA Editions, 1996.

Cousins, Norman. *Anatomy of An Illness As Perceived by the Patient: Reflections on Healing and Regeneration.* New York: Bantam Books, 1979.

DeSalvo, Louise. *Writing As a Way of Healing: How Telling Our Stories Transforms Our Lives.* Boston: Beacon Press. 1999.

———. "How Telling Our Stories Transforms Our Lives." *Poets and Writers Magazine* (May–June 2001): 48–50.

Dove, Rita. "Dawn Revisited." *Callaloo* 2, no. 1 (1999): 24.

Driskill, Joseph. *Protestant Spiritual Exercises: Theology, History and Practice.* Harrisburg, Pa.: Morehouse Publishing, 1999.

Erickson, Tiffany. "Star Coulbrooke: Writing Makes Good Medicine in Women's Lives." *Hard News Café.* Utah State University Department of Journalism and Communications, June 5, 2003.

Felman, Shoshana, and Dori Laub. *Testimony: Crises of Witnessing in Literature, Psychoanalysis and History.* New York: Routledge, 1992.

Foster, Patricia, and Mary Swander, eds. *The Healing Circle: Authors Writing of Recovery.* New York: Plume Books, 1998.

Fox, John. *Poetic Medicine.* New York: Jeremy P. Tarcher/Putnam, 1997.

———. "Recovering Your Silenced Voice." *Poets and Writers Magazine* (May–June 2001): 63–66.

Frank, Arthur W. *The Wounded Storyteller: Body Illness and Ethics.* Chicago: The University of Chicago Press, 1995.

Gallagher, Tess. "The Poem as a Reservoir for Grief." In *A Concert of Tenses.* Ann Arbor: The University of Michigan Press, 1987.

Georgiou, Elena. *Mercy Mercy Me.* Madison: The University of Wisconsin Press, 2000.

Gergen, Kenneth J., and Mary M. Gergen. "Narrative Form and the Construction of Psychological Theory." In T. S. Sarbin, ed., *Narrative Psychology: The Storied Nature of Human Conduct.* New York: Praeger, 1986.

Hacker, Marilyn. *Winter Numbers: Poems*. New York: W. W. Norton, 1994.

Hampl, Patricia. *I Could Tell You Stories: Sojourns in the Land of Memory*. New York: W. W. Norton, 2000.

Henke, Suzette. "Literary Life Writing in the 20th Century." *Poets and Writers Magazine* (May–June 2001): 40–43.

———. *Shattered Subjects*. New York: St. Martin's Press, 1998.

Hikmet, Nazim. *Poems of Nazim Hikmet*. Translated by Randy Blasing and Mutlu Konuk. New York: Persea Books, 1994.

Hoffman, Alice. "Sustained by Fiction While Facing Life's Facts." *The New York Times*, August 14, 2000.

Kinnell, Galway. "St. Francis and the Sow." In *Mortal Acts, Mortal Words*. Boston: Houghton Mifflin, 1960.

Lepore, Stephen J., and Joshua M. Smyth, eds. *The Writing Cure: How Expressive Writing Promotes Health and Well-Being*. Washington D.C.: American Psychological Association, 2002.

Lerner, Michael. "Healing." In *Healing and The Mind*. Edited by Bill Moyers, Sue Flowers, and David Grubin. New York: Doubleday, 1993.

Levine, Philip. "Silent in America." In *New Selected Poems*. New York: Alfred A. Knopf, 2002.

Lorde, Audrey. *The Cancer Journals*. New York: Spinsters Ink, 1980.

Lorden, Lisa. "Writing Is Good Medicine." *CFIDS/Fibromyalgia Self-Help*, April 1, 2003.

MacCurdy, Marian. "Writing and Healing." *Ithaca College Quarterly* 2 (2002). www.ithaca.edu/publication/icq/2000v2/lastlook.htm.

Martin, Chia. *Writing Your Way Through Cancer*. Prescott, Ariz.: Hohm Press, 2000.

Mayer, Musa. "Scribbling My Way to Spiritual Well-Being." *MAMM Magazine* (April 2000): 26–29.

McCarriston, Linda. *Eva Mary*. Evanston, Ill.: TriQuarterly Books, 1991.

Metzger, Deena. *Writing for Your Life: Discovering the Story of Your Life's Journey*. San Francisco: Harper, 1992.

Mitchell, Felicia. "Frances Driscoll and the Rape Poems." *Poets and Writers Magazine* (May–June 2001): 43–47.

Murray, Bridget. "Writing to Heal." *Monitor on Psychology* 33, no. 6 (June 2002). www.apa.org/monitor/jun02/writing.htm

Murray, Kevin. "Life As Fiction." *Journal for the Theory of Social Behavior* 15, no. 2 (1995): 173–88.

Myers, Art, and Maria Marrocchino. *Winged Victory: Altered Images: Transcending Breast Cancer.* San Diego: Photographic Gallery of Fine Art, 1996.

Myers, Linda Joy. *Becoming Whole: Writing Your Healing Story.* San Diego: Silver Threads, 2003.

Otis, Lauren. "Poetry in Prisons, Part Two." *Poets and Writers Magazine* (May–June 2001): 58–62.

Pennebaker, James W. "Confronting a Traumatic Event: Toward an Understanding of Inhibition and Disease." *Journal of Abnormal Psychology* 95, no. 3 (1986): 274–81.

———. "Linguistic Predictors of Adaptive Bereavement." *Journal of Personality and Social Psychology* 72 (1997): 864–71.

———. *Opening Up: The Healing Power of Expressing Emotions.* New York: The Guilford Press, 1997.

———. "Writing About Emotional Experience as a Therapeutic Process." *Psychological Science* 8, no. 3 (1997): 162–66.

Pennebaker, James W., and Jane D. Segal. "Forming a Story: The Health Benefits of Narrative." *Journal of Clinical Psychology* 55, no. 10 (1999): 1243–54.

Remen, Rachel Naomi. "Wholeness." In *Healing and The Mind.* Edited by Bill Moyers, Sue Flowers, and David Grubin. New York: Doubleday, 1993.

Rico, Gabrielle. *Pain and Possibility: Writing Your Way through Personal Crisis.* New York: J. P. Tarcher/Putnam, 1991.

Ridgeway, Leslie, and Dale Griffith. "Struggles: Writing as Healing." *Focus on Basics, Literacy and Health* 5, issue C (February 2002). www.gsu.harvard.edu/~ncsall/fob/2002/ridgway.htm

Roberts, Larenda. "Writing for Their Lives." *Palo Alto Weekly,* November 14, 2001.

Schneider, Pat. *Tell Me Something I Can't Forget: Low Income Women Write about Their Lives.* Video. Produced by Diane Garey and Larry Hott. Florentine Films, 1993.

———. *The Writer As an Artist: Writing Alone and with Others.* Los Angeles: Lowell House, 1993.

———. *Writing Alone and with Others.* New York: Oxford University Press, 2003.

———. *Writing Alone and with Others: A Companion Piece to the Book.* DVD. Produced by Diane Garey and Larry Hott. Florentine Films, 2003.

Schön, Donald. *The Reflective Practitioner: How Professionals Think in Action.* New York: Basic Books, 1983.

Slocombe, Daphne, ed. *What I Had To Say: Writing Groups That Heal. Amherst Writers & Artists Leaders on the Passion and Practice of Their Work.* Amherst, Mass.: Amherst Writers & Artists Press, forthcoming, 2004.

Smyth, J. M., A. A. Stone, A. Hurewitz, and A. Kaell. "Effects of Writing About Stressful Experiences On Symptom Reduction in Patients with Asthma or Rheumatoid Arthritis: A Randomized Trial." *JAMA* (April 14, 1999): 1328.

Smyth, Joshua M. "Writing Your Feelings: Good Medicine for Chronic Conditions." *Habit,* Health Behavior News Service, Center for the Advancement of Health. April 13, 1999.

Sontag, Susan. *Illness as Metaphor.* New York: Farrar, Straus and Giroux, 1978.

———. "The Risk Taker, An Interview with Gary Younge." *The Guardian,* January 19, 2002.

Spiegel, D., J. R. Bloom, H. C. Kraemar, and E. Gottheil. "Effect of Psychosocial Treatment on Survival of Patients with Metastatic Breast Cancer." *Lancet* 2 (1989): 888–91.

Spiegel, D., J. R. Bloom, and I. Yalom. "Group Support for Patients With Metastatic Cancer." *Archives of General Psychiatry* 28, no. 5 (1981): 527–33.

Spiegel, David. *Living beyond Limits.* New York: Ballantine Books, 1993.

———. "Therapeutic Support Groups." In *Healing and The Mind.* Edited by Bill Moyers, Sue Flowers, and David Grubin. New York: Doubleday, 1993.

Spiegel, David, and Catherine Classen. *Group Therapy for Cancer Patients: A Research-based Handbook of Psychosocial Care.* New York: Basic Books, 2000.

Stafford, William. *Crossing Unmarked Snow: Further Views on the Writer's Vocation.* Ann Arbor: The University of Michigan Press, 1997.

———. *You Must Revise Your Life.* Ann Arbor: The University of Michigan Press, 1986.

Stanton, Annette L., Sharon Danoff-Burg, Christine L. Cameron, Michelle Bishop, Charlotte A. Collins, Sarah B. Kirk, and Lisa A Sworowski. "Emotionally Expressive Coping Predicts Psychological and Physical Adjustment to Breast Cancer." *Journal of Consulting and Clinical Psychology* 68, no. 5 (2000): 875–82.

Stanton, Annette L., Sharon Danoff-Burg, Lisa A. Sworowski, Charlotte A. Collins, Ann D. Branstetter, Alicia Rodriguez-Hanley, Sarah B. Kirk, and Jennifer L. Austenfeld. "Randomized, Controlled Trial of Written Emotional Expression and Benefit Finding in Breast Cancer Patients." *Journal of Clinical Oncology* 20, no. 20 (2002): 4160–68.

Stegner, Wallace. *On Teaching and Writing Fiction*. New York: Penguin Books, 2002.

Stoltz, Ron. "The White Rat Talks Back." Personal communication, 1986.

Stromberg, Sandi. "Mind Matters: Scientists Study the Impact of Expressive Writing on Cancer." *Network Newsletter*, a publication of the Anderson Network, The University of Texas, M. D. Anderson Cancer Center, 2002.

Taylor, Daniel. *The Healing Power of Stories: Creating Yourself from the Stories of Your Life*. New York: Bantam Books, 1996.

Vecchione, Patrice. *Writing and the Spiritual Life: Finding Your Voice by Looking Within*. New York: McGraw Hill/Contemporary Books, 2001.

Vega, Janine. "Poetry in Prisons, Part One." *Poets and Writers Magazine* (May–June, 2001): 56–58.

Ventling, Christina D. "Epilogue: Writing As Healing." In C. D. Ventling, ed., *Body Psychotherapy in Progressive and Chronic Disorders*. Basel: Karger, 2002.

Zimmerman, Susan. *Writing to Heal the Soul: Transforming Grief and Loss through Writing*. New York: Three Rivers Press, 2001.